Myofascial Magic in Action

of related interest

Yoga, Fascia, Anatomy and Movement, Second Edition
Joanne Avison
ISBN 978 1 91342 604 0
eISBN 978 1 91342 605 7

Spiral Bound
Integrated Anatomy for Yoga
Karen Kirkness
ISBN 978 1 91208 503 3
eISBN 978 1 91208 504 0

Fascia in Sport and Movement, Second Edition
Edited by Robert Schleip, Jan Wilke, and Amanda Baker
Foreword by Thomas W Findley
ISBN 978 1 91208 577 4
eISBN 978 1 91208 578 1

Scars, Adhesions and the Biotensegral Body
Science, Assessment and Treatment
Edited by Jan Trewartha and Sharon Wheeler
Forewords by Robert Schleip and Carol M Davis
ISBN 978 1 91208 546 0
eISBN 978 1 91208 547 7

Architecture of Human Living Fascia
The Extracellular Matrix and Cells Revealed Through Endoscopy
Jean-Claude Guimberteau and Colin Armstrong
Forewords by Thomas W Findley and Adalbert I Kapandji
ISBN 978 1 80501 257 3
eISBN 978 1 80501 308 2

MYOFASCIAL MAGIC IN ACTION

A Movement Practitioner's Guide to How the Body Really Moves

Dr Joanne Avison

Illustrated by Dr Joanne Avison
Foreword by John Sharkey

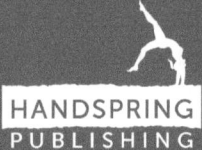

HANDSPRING
PUBLISHING

First published in Great Britain in 2025 by Handspring Publishing,
an imprint of Jessica Kingsley Publishers
Part of John Murray Press

2

A CIP catalogue record for this title is available from the
British Library and the Library of Congress

ISBN 978 1 83997 775 6
eISBN 978 1 83997 776 3

Printed and bound in the UK by Ashford Colour Ltd.

Jessica Kingsley Publishers' policy is to use papers that are natural,
renewable and recyclable products and made from wood grown in
sustainable forests. The logging and manufacturing processes are expected
to conform to the environmental regulations of the country of origin.

Handspring Publishing
Carmelite House
50 Victoria Embankment
London EC4Y 0DZ

www.handspringpublishing.com

John Murray Press
Part of Hodder & Stoughton Limited
An Hachette UK Company

This book is dedicated to my spiritual teacher John-Roger, with love and light.

Contributors

HELEN EADIE

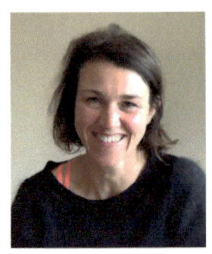

Helen is deeply curious about the relationship between body consciousness and mind, specifically how we can heal psychological wounds through the body's process of becoming conscious of itself. She has been a practitioner of craniosacral therapy since 2011, has taught yoga (inspired by the approach of Vanda Scravelli) and somatic movement since 2014, holds a master's degree in psychology from the University of Sussex, and is applying for a psychology research PhD in 2024 to study how somatic practices can support body image, disordered eating and exercise dependence. Between studying and practicing, her favourite things to do are hang out with her family and friends and get a daily dose of nature, either sea swimming or walking across the South Downs with her cocker spaniel.

WILBOUR KELSICK

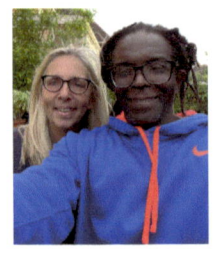

Dr Wilbour Kelsick is the founder and spiritual core of the MaxFit Movement Institute. He has been working as medical staff with the Canadian National and Olympic teams for over 26 years. He also served with the NHL, the NBA and attended 10 Olympic Games as a health practitioner. In addition, he has been a sports medicine consultant with Olympic athletes from the USA, Africa, the Caribbean, and Sweden to name a few. His education and experience position him perfectly for this role. Dr Kelsick's network of colleagues and friends, gathered in his more than 30 years as a healthcare practitioner, expands what he can offer. Dr Kelsick received his BSc in kinesiology from Simon Fraser University and his doctor of chiropractic medicine degree from the Canadian Memorial Chiropractic College.

KAREN KIRKNESS

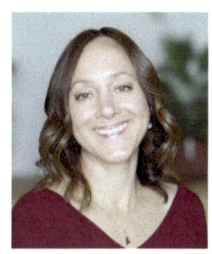

Dr Karen Kirkness is the author of *Spiral Bound: Integrated Anatomy for Yoga* and founder of Meadowlark Yoga in Edinburgh, Scotland. Karen is a busy mother of two and an E-RYT 500 teacher, offering CPD as a committed movement educator passionate about facilitating healthy outcomes through guided self-practice. Originally an Ashtangi, Karen has been practicing yoga since the late 1990s. She has coined her approach to human biomechanics as the Five Filaments, a spiral motion rubric making sense of coupled joint coordination such as the scapulohumeral rhythm. Karen holds an MFA and MSc in human anatomy, as well as a doctorate of philosophy in medical sciences with a focus on anatomy pedagogy and complexity theory in the UK medical curriculum.

JOHN SHARKEY

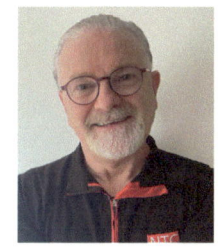

John Sharkey, MSc, is an accredited clinical anatomist, member of the Anatomical Society (AS) and British Association of Clinical Anatomists (BACA). He is an international educator, author, and recognized authority in the areas of clinical anatomy, fascia science, human movement, and the treatment of myofascial pain. John is a graduate of the University of Dundee, University of Liverpool, and University of Chester. He completed studies in the areas of exercise physiology and clinical anatomy and holds a postgraduate certificate in education from Maynooth University, Ireland. John is the programme leader of the biotensegrity-focused cadaver dissection courses that have been held at the University of Dundee, King's College London, The Ohio State University, Trecchi Human, Italy, and internationally.

PAUL THORNLEY

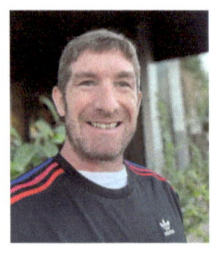

Paul is originally from Manchester, England where he began studying Karate from the age of seven. At 19, he joined the Royal Airforce, supporting pilots on their flight missions. In places like Saudi Arabia, Paul's physical strength was challenged to the limit and he learned the hard way how to respond quickly and resiliently to those challenges.

In his 30's, with enormous respect for the human body, Paul changed careers to study the body in even more depth. He became a Neuro-Muscular Therapist to understand manual therapy and trained with STOTT Pilates, eventually becoming a top movement Instructor Trainer in Dubai and then around the world.

Paul's studies and dedication to the wholeness of the human body and how the entire fascia matrix works under stress and rest brought him to studying human dissection, movement, and rehab with world-renowned specialists. His deep understanding of Myofascia and Fasciategrity is revealed in his unique delivery and practical presentations.

Contents

Foreword

John Sharkey, MSc

Enter a realm where the mundane meets the mystical, where the ordinary transforms into the extraordinary, and where the essence of being transcends the confines of mere mechanics. Pinocchio is a classic Italian children's novel about a wooden puppet who dreams of becoming a real boy. The wooden puppet yearns to transcend his mechanical constraints as humanity too grapples with the notion of transcending its mechanistic existence. *Myofascial Magic in Action* by Joanne Avison beautifully captures this essence, offering a transformative account that guides us toward a deeper understanding of our unified being. Just like a machine, Pinocchio is made of the wrong 'stuff' and is pinned together to create limbs that move. He has no breath, no blood coursing through his veins. Metaphorically speaking, the 400 year-old definition of man as machine means we are all Pinocchio, and *Myofascial Magic in Action* gifts all of us with our wish to, at last, be whole and unified.

In *Myofascial Magic in Action*, Joanne Avison takes us on a profound journey of rediscovery, a journey that illuminates the unified body, mind, and spirit through a lens of metaphorical exploration. With Joanne's signature blend of wisdom and whimsy, she deftly unravels centuries-old 'puppet like' misconceptions surrounding the human body, guiding us toward a deeper understanding of our innate wholeness. Through the enchanting medium of cartoon characters and exquisite use of language, Joanne breathes life into these pages, as only she can, inviting readers of all ages to embark on an adventure of self-discovery and transformation.

Using the captivating narrative of metaphor, a bridge that carries us from the realm of abstract ideas to the realm of embodied experience, Avison skilfully navigates the terrain, revealing how metaphor shapes our perception of movement, medicine, and the very essence of our being. In her hands, metaphor becomes a tool for liberation, a catalyst for expanding our awareness and embracing the full spectrum of human expression. Drawing upon her deep well of knowledge and insight, Avison challenges us to reconsider the outdated paradigms that have long confined our understanding of the body. Through her insightful guidance, we are encouraged to embrace a more holistic perspective, one that celebrates the inherent magic of our existence and honours the intricate dance of life within us all. There is no need for a puppeteer pulling strings for us to be or be moved.

As we journey through these pages we are reminded of the profound wisdom encoded within the very fabric of our being. Avison's words resonate with a clarity and depth that transcends the limitations of language, inviting us to reawaken to the innate wonder that resides within each of us. With a blend of humour, insight, and profound wisdom, *Myofascial Magic in Action* transcends from a book to a beacon of light guiding each of us home to ourselves. Joanne embarks on a courageous exploration of the very foundations upon which our understanding of anatomy and movement has been built.

With a keen eye for detail and a profound reverence for the mysteries of the human body, Joanne dares to ask the questions that have long lingered in the shadows of conventional wisdom. 'What if we discovered that all we've been learning about anatomy these last 400 years is based on a metaphor that is, simply, wrong?' Avison challenges us to confront this startling possibility head-on, inviting us to re-evaluate the very essence of our existence. In doing so, Joanne opens the door to a world where the mundane and the magical intertwine, where the rigid confines of mechanistic 'Pinocchio-style thinking' give way to the boundless creativity of the human spirit.

Through her meticulous research and heartfelt reflections, Avison sheds light on the tangled web of metaphors that have shaped our understanding of the body and its intricate workings. From the mechanical paradigm of the Industrial Revolution to the architectural symbolism of the Renaissance, Avison traces the evolution of these metaphors and their profound impact on our perception of ourselves.

Yet amidst the shadows of misconception, Avison reveals a glimmer of hope, a beacon of light illuminating the path toward a more holistic and integrated understanding of the human body. With each turn of the page, she challenges us to embrace the innate magic of our existence, to celebrate the unique tapestry of our beingness, and to awaken to the boundless potential that resides within each of us. As we journey through this rich tapestry we are reminded of the profound interconnectedness of all things, the delicate dance of life that unfolds within and around us. With her trademark blend of insight and inspiration, Joanne Avison invites us to reclaim our birthright as conscious, embodied beings, to rediscover the joy of movement, the wonder of expression, and the infinite possibilities that lie within the depths of our being.

So, dear reader, let us embark on this transformative journey together, as we unravel the mysteries of the human body and awaken to the magic that resides within us all. For in the words of Joanne Avison, 'Everyone is already a dancer' and it is time to dance with life in all its glorious complexity. 'To-morrow I cease to be a puppet, and I become a boy like you and all the other boys' (Pinocchio).

With much love, light and gratitude to Joanne for her spirit of sharing.

John Sharkey
Clinical Anatomist, Exercise Physiologist
Dublin, Ireland, 2025

Acknowledgements

My deepest gratitude and thanks to all my family, my ministerial family, my 'friend families', my 'work families', and the families I love and work with all around the world.

You know who you are, I love you, thank you and appreciate you,

Joanne,
Brighton, 2024

Introduction

AWAKENING TO WHAT ALREADY IS: HOW *MYOFASCIAL MAGIC IN ACTION* EMERGED

Myofascial Magic in Action was born out of many years of practice, even more years of study, and a short course that emerged during lockdown in response to a lot of questions! The questions arose from several sources: the anatomy laboratory, the yoga classroom, the manual therapy classroom, my clinical practice, the fascinating world of conferences (as delegate and presenter), and over 25 years of working with the moving body as movement teacher and manual practitioner. There were lots of responses to my first book, *Yoga, Fascia, Anatomy and Movement* – and then more from the second edition. *Myofascial Magic in Action* grew out of all of that.

As an artist, originally, I was completely fascinated by body and movement patterns. When I began teaching movement, nearly 30 years ago, I diligently learned the origins and insertions of muscles, the biomechanics of levers and the stories of how the spine moves as an upright inverted pendulum. It made little sense of the moving beings in my classrooms.

At the end of 1998 (so last century!), I began working with Tom Myers, proofreading the original first edition of Anatomy Trains™ (AT). I eventually became one of his early teachers, at times sleeping on a mattress on the floor of his study, surrounded by the books *he* had studied to write about the continuities of the body's so-called myofascial meridians. They made more sense of living body movement than the 'body bits' I had learned from the anatomy atlas. After working with AT for several years, I established the keys to using the continuities of these 'body bands' in motion. It is a very particular way of working with them, that I taught in Pilates and yoga schools in the 'noughties' and eventually my own yoga teacher training in 2008. Yet they still didn't answer certain questions from the movement classroom – they didn't explain the unique expression of each version of a pose, by the unique being that performed it at the time. Manual therapy of structural integration gave me even more insight into the individuality of each person I met or had the privilege to work with. Tom once told me that I needed 15 clients a week, for five years, to truly sense what was going on in a body through my hands. It felt like forever at the three-year mark – and 25 years later, I know what it takes to become a 'fascia whisperer'. That granted me the wisdom to teach touch skills to movement teachers and transform them into movement mentors.

It was a series of shocks and light bulb moments that woke me up to what is really the difficulty and the difference in teaching movement – for all of us – that *Myofascial Magic in Action* seeks to resolve. Let me briefly share what those keystone moments were:

Shock number 1

I was present at the first human dissection programme to establish the AT – and there was my first shock. Namely that the 'train lines' had been deduced from an idea, from the intellectual study of muscles and bones – not the lab. In the anatomy laboratory, not only are there no lines, but those so-called 'trains' don't work the same or appear in the same way in all bodies. That is where I learned my first vital lesson in making a difference to other people's movement patterns. That lesson was loud and clear: *one size does not fit all*. One anatomy does not explain all, one body in the anatomy book does not represent all. One line does not say it all. Not at all.

Shock number 2

Movement is not an intellectual process and it cannot be reduced to one, however good we are with words. We need metaphors, and the AT was one such metaphor. It retained the 'mechanical' part of the movement equation and took us from the classical anatomy of 'biomechanical bits' into the contemporary anatomy of 'biomechanical bands'.

That is a great step forward and it would be complete if they made sense of every body and every movement. They do and they don't. They are a superbly useful segue into considering the body as related, organized, and in continuity from ground to crown. However, they keep us stuck considering slings as if they exist (especially if we forget it is a metaphor). And here was my second shock when working with actual bodies: without question or exception, the AT were carved, not revealed.

Every body is unique and whole and relentlessly continuous, in all directions, anyway.

EVERY BODY IS UNIQUE! Professor Darrel Evans, at Brighton and Sussex Medical School, endorsed that for me later and upgraded my understanding of anatomy. Years of working with clinical anatomist John Sharkey since then, and Associate Professor of Anatomy and Embryology, Jaap van der Val, have added the confirmation of their generous teachings in anatomy and embryology of the fascia.

Shock number 3

The AT form a fascinating foundation to a journey moving from classical bits to contemporary bands. They proved a super helpful metaphor when recognizing movement patterns, when you know how to work with the AT metaphor in practice. However, this train journey doesn't get us from bands to bodies. It falls way short of representing your so-called 'anatomy trains, planes and automobility' as uniquely expressed by you; the whole being that resides in your entirely and invariably unique body! YOU are the driver of the train, the tracks and the territory you build them on. You grew all of it yourself. AS A WHOLE. The wholeness came first.

That was shock number three! The unique spirit (that in living beings would animate the whole form as a whole) was 'present as missing' in the anatomy laboratory. In other words, it had no living matter through which to express itself. Yet historically, we base many conclusions about how the living body self-organizes, thinks and feels on something that is essentially cut out from the dead body.

It was wonderfully useful to learn from, but it had no say in the *matter of living motion*. YOU have a say in that, every moment of every day with every breath you take and every move you make. That's your power and your grace, to change your form in motion moment to moment. It is the sign of life.

My journey with Tom and AT is one I treasure, with all its difficulties and steep learning curves. It was enlightening and demanding on every level. It raised my game and the number of questions I had to ask. It brought me, inexorably, to working with Dr Caroline Myss at the CMED Institute to better understand the being, that was 'present as missing' in the laboratory of bodies. I studied Sacred Contracts in person with Caroline, over several years, learning archetypal patterns of the psyche and becoming a practitioner in the field of medical intuition. It fascinated me, and I returned to my practice, staying bound to the physical and the literal in my movement classroom and structural integration clinic. Transforming these three shocks into guiding principle questions kept me practising, curious, and asking more questions.

I resolved to understand how we *really* move. Does the archetypal pattern of the beings that danced around me reflect or impact the bodies they animated? Could knowing that make a difference? If so, how could it be translated into practice – *for everyone?*

Light bulb moment number 1

What I discovered, over a period of 25 years, is that the archetypal nature of our psyche (meaning soul) is not separate or different from the fabric of our human form. It can seem distinct; however, it shares its manner and its mannerisms. Fascia is archetypal too. The congruency we are all trained to foster in mind and emotion, can actually be found between body and being – once we understand that they were never separate in the first place. When I realized that the fascia matrix is archetypal – unique to each one of us – my first 'great big huge' (as Caroline Myss would say) light bulb moment occurred. Body and being are one, expressed in unique combinations of archetypal patterns. It's what makes us all the same, ironically – we are all invariably unique.[1]

Light bulb moment number 2

Then I realized my body doesn't speak English (or any of our 'mother tongues'). I realized it speaks in sensations and the way I interpret them; it depends on which archetypes I'm listening to and what meaning I assign to them. That was light bulb moment number two.

---

1   Archetypes, according to the definition presented by Carl Jung, suggest primitive patterns of human behaviour (inherited) that are deep to the collective unconscious. However, in this sense we are considering the work of more modern philosophers, such as Dr Caroline Myss (as one of many examples), where these patterns are described and recognized in practical ways as something of a guiding template of the true personality. As such, it could be said, that each person has 'key traits' that make up the unique coordinates of their individual archetypal nature.

Light bulb moment number 3

The third light bulb moment was realizing that for all the scientific rea-soning and scientific researchers seeking to 'stereotype' the fascia matrix into its component parts, to name each one of them and find out if it's a 'thing' or a 'system', or how to describe it formally in the light of fascia research, it's never going to fit.

You are the architect that self-organized your architecture to express yourself as the architect.

That was my 'mic drop', magical, nothing-will-ever-be-the-same-again realization that changed my life permanently and left me stunned, curious, and very isolated. We self-organize our living archetypal archi-tecture to express our living selves in Earth School. It's really stating the obvious in many ways – and that is precisely where the significance of the Fascia Matrix has been hiding for four centuries. Right there in plain sight, enfolded in the obvious, where we missed it.

AN ARCHETYPAL COLLECTIVE

Fortunately, I wasn't alone for long. After a few years of questions, study, conferences, reading research papers, and diligently teaching and treat-ing people every week to get the experience in my hands (they speak fluent fascia in numerous dialects, just through practicing), I found myself part of an amazing team of people to work with.

I'm fortunate enough to have met some incredible beings, besides my team. Professors and practitioners; doctors and dancers; movement, medical, and manual therapists; surgeons and specialists; researchers and Reiki masters; scientists and spiritual leaders; publishers and peers; authors and entrepreneurs; ministers and mavens; chocolatiers and charlatans; friends and family. Every one of them has contributed to my story and although some taught me by default (i.e., what *not* to do), most taught me by design what can really work and why it makes a difference in the world. The majority are as curious as I am, so between us we never stop learning and sharing our collective questions and discoveries.

That is the foundation upon which this series of books stands at this point in time.

THE UNPREDICTABLE POSSIBILITIES

During the pandemic years, in the 2020s, like many, I had to pivot and respond to some of the questions I was asked after writing *Yoga, Fascia, Anatomy and Movement.* I used 'yoga' in the title to give me access to referencing spirit in a semi-academic book that really applies to all movement modalities. This book sought to bring together much of the fascia research into a story that could shift us from thinking about the body as separate from the being and made of disconnected parts. It took a journey towards seeing the fascia differently as a whole unified structure, that communicates in sound, light and biomotional sensation – I call it biomotional intelligence. It's an orchestra that we aren't even aware of some of the time. It hums its symphony to the sound of nature's exquisite Unstruck Chord.[2]

Now I have more courage and confidence, as a reverend and a doctor of spiritual science, having studied Surat Shabd yoga for nearly a decade. I dare to consider the fascia matrix as the interface of spirit (or consciousness) animating our form. The soul resides in the soma (or the soma in the soul). The body in the being (or the being in the body). They don't have anywhere else to go. We are one – whatever we think – it's inclusive, naturally. The fascia is our forming fabric – and we self-organize into form as embryos.

Myofascial Magic in Action was the first of several masterclasses I designed during lockdown and taught online; partly because I was asked to and partly because there was no other way to do it! Post pandemic and post becoming very ill soon after, I used my own learning and teaching experiences to recover. I brought the archetypal artist back into my energy field and by coincidence or design, my new publisher saw the sketches. Her delight brought this first book, in a series of five, into being. I hope the drawings somehow animate the text so you can enjoy discovering all that helped me to recover and continue to restore my health and well-being. My bigger hope is that it serves you to serve many others.

My publisher asked me to turn each Masterclass into a book that was easy to read and put into action, with the story of the myofascial matrix

---

2   The Anahata Nad refers to the sound of the Unstruck Chord. It is the basis of Surat Shabd yoga.

as an asset to movement. Here is the first of the series and it is written, by design, in an easy, accessible voice without dense referencing or much attempt at semi-academic standards of literature. It draws heavily on the information in *Yoga, Fascia, Anatomy and Movement* (which has been updated in the second edition) and you can go there for more details and further references. In the meantime, through all this study and work, I have completed nearly a decade of learning to become a minister and study spiritual science, as a background to all the above. As Reverend Dr Avison, I have seen and studied – in depth – how 'doing does it' and my deep bias is towards the beautiful inspiration Dr Paul Kaye gave me back in 2015. His question, regarding understanding fascia, was, 'How does it help me move better?'

That question leads each one of these books, and I write them in service and devotion to every movement teacher out there, dedicated to serving those they teach. I rarely meet one who isn't devoted and heart-centred in their earnest desire to make a difference to others. It is to and for you that I write and share these ideas. It is for you that Paul Thornley and I created the course that accompanies the book, if you are inspired to go deep and acquire these skills directly.

This book is practical and focused on myofascial magic and the 'in action' bit that brings it forth. It isn't biased to any particular movement modality. However, with my colleague, Paul Thornley, who has devoted his work to the Pilates field, we have created a course to show you how to animate the practices this book explains and presents.

Before we begin, however, we must understand one of the keystones in our consciousness, that allows us to understand anything. That keystone is metaphor. It is super important, and we will begin there, in Part 1. Once we understand which metaphors have us spellbound and how we might upgrade them, we go practical.

In the introduction to Volume 1 in his brilliant work *The Matter with Things,* Iain McGilchrist wrote:

> *...specialization makes it even harder to expect more than a tiny handful of scientists and philosophers to be in a position to venture into a genuinely new understanding of their (in reality) common enterprise, one that has the potential hugely to enrich both parties. When any attempt is made to reach out a hand across the distancing void, it is almost invariably an exercise in reinforcing the status quo:*

*the scientists telling the philosophers that they find only machines,
and the philosophers reflecting back to the scientists that a mechanistic view is the best option on offer. Since what you find is a product
of how you attend, this is a more or less pointless exercise in making
sure that both parties sink to the bottom in the shortest possible time.*

With the support of an exceptional number of brilliant and dedicated
professionals, scientists and philosophers as well as practitioners (each
outstanding in their own field), this work is hallmarked by its focus away
from a mechanistic view. I feel very privileged to be 'on team' in the
laboratory with some of these people – and on the phone to others! It's
a stunning collective and in no way decreases the value and appreciation
of all those in the acknowledgements.

The team members include John Sharkey, Paul Thornley, Dr Wilbour
Kelsick, Mark Flannigan, Dr Karen Kirkness, Helen Eadie, Bex Hawkins,
Mark Jubber, Lisa Babiuk, Michelle Martin, Vic Evans, Shane McDermott,
Ben Avison, Deborah Martinez, Kate Dooley, Michelle van Straaten,
Maria do Carmo, Oonagh Brown, Jo Cruikshank, and many others. My
close ties to several senior professionals in the health science field and
gorgeous humans who keep me focused and in service, are all involved
in this work. These books include their contributions and we work (as
we all can) as a collective. Each focused on our own speciality and each
working towards making the emergent properties of this work – as a
whole – greater than the sum of its parts. That's how our bodies work
and how this body of work emerges.

My gratitude is great, big, huge. My intention is that you can make
a bigger difference to those you already make a difference to – serving
them even better with this knowledge threaded into the tapestry of
whatever movement teaching and learning you already weave.

May it bless many.

Part 1

THE HISTORY

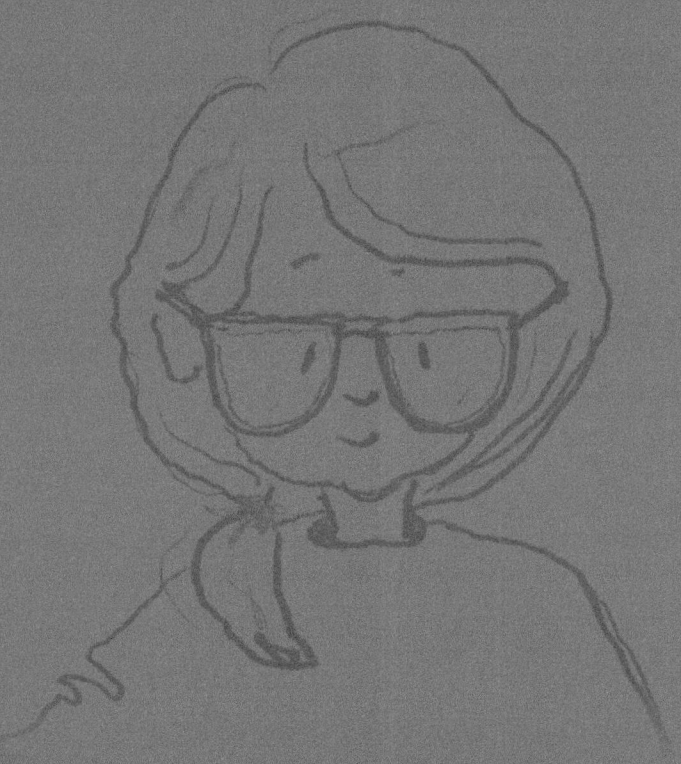

THE MATTER AND THE METAPHOR

Something as big as a cultural history...as big as politics...as big as a religion...as big as the basis of the physical sciences...has divorced the being from the body for 400 years. Something bigger is transforming that cultural conditioning within each one of us. Something that taught us our body parts are 'separate, mechanical and need uniting in order to be embodied' is now (somehow) remembering that we begin whole and complete and create and weave and organize those parts, from within the wholeness. Our selves. We begin whole and complete. We live that way. We continue whole and complete. We live and complete our lives that way. We simply forget. Something beyond description is guiding us to recognize that the very same intention (to understand and serve humans being) is retransforming our separate factions and body parts back into the wholeness, the unique collective, that they always already are.

AWAKENING TO THE POWER OF METAPHOR

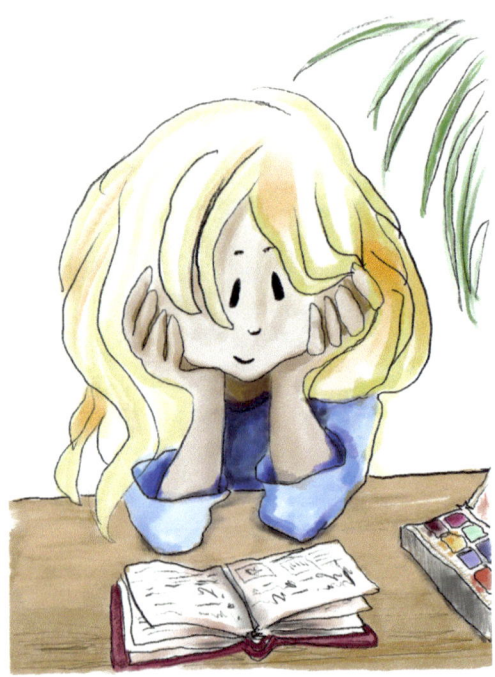

Figure 1

The definition of metaphor is *meta* – meaning across + *pherein* – meaning to carry. The purpose of metaphor is to 'carry us across' from an idea to an embodied experience. Metaphor is so deep to our everyday language that like the fascia of the human form, it's hidden in the obvious. Perhaps it is hard to realize how much we use metaphor in speech, imagery, and the written word, to provide meaning and understanding.

Metaphor literally has the power to 'carry' us across from the darkness of not knowing to the brightness of understanding, the *enlightenment* that expands our awareness. The problem is that metaphors can often be so overused, that they are collapsed with reality. A metaphor points towards similarity and uncanniness, but it is not a synonym, *meaning it is not the same as the thing it describes or allows us to experience*. Its purpose is to inspire a breakthrough in perception, unlike the standard use of language which is more focused with representing reality literally. Metaphor provides a kind of symbolism that can shape our experience.

When it comes to understanding the human body and how it moves, modern movement, manual and medical therapies operate under particular metaphors. In many cases, it isn't even obvious that they've been lost in translation and somehow misrepresented the actual experience, for centuries.

The metaphor in which the study of human motion lives is that of the machine. When 'mechanics' is the foundational term used to describe the living, moving, human body; it demonstrates how metaphor and meaning can become collapsed. Despite how modern technology can now see inside the body in unprecedented ways, the old metaphor, from 400 years ago, is still in use. It is worth considering how this mechanical foundation has formed our understanding and approach to ourselves in terms of how we move and even how we 'be'. In some ways it has cut us off from the very expression each one of us naturally inherits.

We each express our beingness through movement – it is the essence of life, and it is essentially the gestures each one of us performs in our own way that make me into me and you into you and them into them. Everyone has a unique 'body language'; a way of incorporating their eccentricities and ways *to express themselves*. For the centuries that the machine has been used as the founding metaphor, that knowledge (or gnosis) has been elusive. In some ways it is as if the healing arts are somehow 'less than' medicine, for considering there is much more to 'human being' than mechanical reference and reliance on linear, data-based information.

This part will go deep and compassionately on how the wrong metaphors arose in our history. It's essential to understand the focus of the founding fathers of modern science to appreciate (and evolve) our understanding beyond their knowledge, without excluding it. We can respectfully maintain a forgiving understanding of the history of human anatomy, without holding on to the idea that mind–body–spirit are separate categories within us, once the circumstances under which medicine began are understood. If we are to restore wholeness and reconnect with the natural inner wisdom from which we self-organized in the first place, it may be of enormous benefit to find new metaphors to enhance how the learning and teaching of movement happens. It is, after all, the basis of living expression. How do we incorporate our experience and enjoy it, rather than analyse it and live in the gaps between the data and the dance? Everyone is already a dancer.

THE MACHINE

I will repeat this frequently. You are not a machine. Neither am I. Neither is anyone. Not one single living *anything* on this planet is mechanical like a clock or a car or washing machine. By definition we are all *non-linear biologic forms – whole (conscious) ones at that.* That means, in the simplest language, not one of us begins with a mechanical part, nor are we made from them, when we are born. It also means we have no lines, levers, stacked bones, exact symmetries, flat planes, right angles or bolts or pins or screws or frames or lights or plumbing or wiring or hard-matter forms in us anywhere in our original structure.

It is the wrong metaphor *for the living*. It is a dead metaphor, and it is like a dead weight around the ankles of the human ability to thrive as essentially spiritual, animated, heart-centred, whole beings – in motion as a sign of life. Each of us does that in a unique archetypal way – there is no one way. Yet medicine and movement and manual therapy rely on generic, one-size-fits-all, mechanical metaphors. Movement is taught and studied on the basis that we are mechanical, and movement forces are described as mechanical forces. It is a metaphor and as Iain McGilchrist suggests (see quotation on p. 21) it ensures we all sink.

Modern technology now allows as different a view of the inner body world as it does of the outer world of the whole cosmos, compared to what was visible from the earliest telescopes and microscopes. Four hundred years ago, the founding fathers of modern medicine and science (and astrological physics) had no such view as can be seen today. They may have *begun* the journey that provided access to the technology modern health enjoys. However, while *their position* and the metaphors they used to help others understand it, made perfect sense to them at the time, it doesn't mean we need to settle for their view as the last word on ours, 400 years later. We have evolved from the Industrial Revolution.

We have satellite navigation in 360 degrees, yet the metaphor of the (mostly) 2D anatomy atlas is still the foundation of how we navigate the territory of the human body. It doesn't work like that – it works more like the cosmos, in 360 degrees. Yet unless we recognize and shift the metaphors, we won't readily be able to imagine ourselves as whole, multidimensional beings within a whole cosmos, with an inner cosmos as fascinating as the one our planet spins us in, much less navigate our way to fully incorporating our embodied selves.

THE RENAISSANCE

In the times of the Industrial Revolution, perhaps it made sense to liken the human body to the mechanical functions of a machine, because machines embraced the best achievements of the day. From the telegraph to the telephone to tomorrow's technology is the story of multiple quantum leaps. These are all the results of tremendous progress that is difficult to appreciate, as each leap has a million marvellous stories of its own. Regardless of the conclusions, or the judgements about them, the facts of how far human progress has come in the last four centuries is phenomenal.

Before the telephone or the car, before the washing machine or the printer, when 'digital' was only an anatomical term for a finger, the word 'bio' was placed in front of 'mechanical' and a story of *metaphorical* human motion was adopted. It was *metaphorically* described as 'biomechanical function'. It has since collapsed into a belief that the body is biomechanical. It can't be – there's no machine here.

The human 'locomotor system' is still studied as if it is based in 'bio-mechanics'. The metaphor somehow morphed into theories that grew factual acceptance, and everyone forgot it was a metaphor in the first place. Academic institutions manufacture that premise and even the more evolved understanding that we 'self-assemble' suggests a production line. We do indeed 'self-assemble' but invariably that is a unique process of living self-organization. It is anything *but* mechanical. Like all fauna, flora and microbiota, it retains certain qualities of the mystical and the magical – it is not mechanical. Reducing biology down into mechanical terms doesn't make human beings into machines.

You and I, us and they, are humans being. That is beings animating bodies (or bodies animating beings, depending on the view). Modern day culture, at least in the West, has been spellbound for centuries by the idea that the mind, the body, and the spirit (not to mention the soul) can be considered separately and the physical aspects of that body being, reduced to the metaphor of a machine *in everyday life*. It is how the body is analysed, assessed, treated and taught – and many movement systems are based upon exercising the individual parts in order to improve how the [body] machine functions. Many trainings work on parts and protocols. *What about the whole magical mystery of each individual form* – the one animating the training?

Essentially, machines are made up of *separate* parts put together in particular ways – the result of which is a given, whole (mechanical) product. But living beings *start* whole and remain that way at all times. This is a very important distinction that sets mechanics and organic, living things apart. Even if, tragically, someone loses a limb – they remain whole in its absence. The limb may be lost, however, *the being is not*. Its body may have changed shape, but it is still a whole being expressing through that body, whatever shape it is in. *As embryos, every single body formed their parts and particularities within the(ir) wholeness.*

> *And that machine thinking comes from the notion that the body is built up from parts. That is the machine-view. That is not true: the embryo shows us loud and clear: First the whole, then the parts. First the matrix, next the elements, first the body, then the organs!!!!!!!!!*
>
> *A machine is built up from parts. That the system might work LIKE a machine does not prove it IS a machine. That you can replace a joint*

*by a hinge does not prove it is a hinge. It works **like** a hinge and that is a big essential difference!!!*

(Jaap van der Wal, Emeritus Associate Professor,
Anatomy and Embryology)[1]

What if we discovered that all we've been learning about anatomy these last 400 years is based on a metaphor that is, simply, wrong? What if the spell needs to be broken so that we can all live much more happily within bodies, embracing the mystery and the magic of our unique experiences? What if we behold only *one* tissue that expresses variation and difference, as distinct from individual, separate parts that are supposed to collectively make us whole? Could it be that if we tune into ourselves enough, we discover that we *store* abilities in our tissue matrix and select and use them as and when we need to in life?

How did the body and the being get so deeply segregated in the first place, that a metaphor of a machine could become the foundation of studying humans moving for *hundreds* of years?

400 YEARS OF RAPID PROGRESS

Four hundred years ago, in the 1620s, even books were rare and hand-written (the first printing press wasn't invented until 1644). Most people couldn't read. Books were reproduced by devoted (and literal) copy writing (as in copying the words into writing by a scribe) that took lifetimes of devotion to complete. Four centuries later there are books, eBooks, and even self-publishing. Modern 'copy writers' are becoming redundant, as artificial intelligence (AI) combines more subtleties, talents, and examples from the masses of information available to the world than anyone could hope to learn in a lifetime with the press of a finger, and a few integrated downloads of data those predecessors could have never imagined.

From handmade ink and a quill pen made out of a bird's feather to this age of technology, where no ink is required, was a powerful transition and transformation. Between those long-gone days of

---

1   Personal communication, July 2013.

diligent (rather than digital) copying and this age of technology was the culture-transforming Industrial Revolution. The predecessors were as fascinated and progressive in their dreams and realizations as their great-great-grandchildren are now – with the caveat that in a few generations time, so much of the current knowledge will have been superseded by our great-great-grandchildren! (I personally pray they will respect their myofascial matrix as a whole expression of themselves and treat it with infinitely more wisdom than is the general norm today!)

The point being made here is that the metaphor of machinery became the basis upon which the human body was studied and learned because it was (back then) the most advanced expression of civilization as mankind could imagine it. The mechanical metaphor was the most progressive available at the time for advancing the study of life itself, including human anatomy and medicine, yet it came with a cost. It separated bodies from beings and analysed one at the expense of the other. (We will go deeper on this shortly).

Indeed, it is not uncommon for doctors to look at scans and data and have no comment on the being they apply to. More expensive perhaps, is the cost of imagining that our performance is based on the practice (e.g., sport) or the goals we achieve (medals and trophies) rather than the experience of ourselves performing. Sometimes everyday life can seem like a marathon. Can we be as captivated by the joy of a gesture, as we are enthralled by first place in a competition? Are minor movements as key to us as major goals?

The cost is essentially the subtle, unique, goal-less power of gesture – the quality, rather than the quantity of results of a being, being themselves, the way they are biomotionally. There's nothing mechanical about *any* body that hasn't been artificially added. Even if that is the language in general use; humans are *not* made of parts, assembled and organized with a manual or by a craftsman. No limbs were bolted on, no sensory organs (or any viscera) were ever inserted and at no time during a pregnancy was any body wired for sound or plugged into a light source or plumbed ready for hydration. Nor did they have 'love' inserted into their functionality as a separate ingredient, or 'awareness' added to their repertoire as if it was purchased like an app on a mobile phone.

Awareness is the foundation of a heart-centred animation of beingness on every level. Like the whole that gave rise to the parts; like the fabric of the form, human becoming is a heart-centred process of revelation that every being undergoes. *Every one.* That treasure was lost to science when it reduced the body down into its parts, as if they could somehow be explained by a theory of how they might be put back together. A theory that no one will ever prove because it is a mystery. Everyone already put themselves together, in order to be here. No one came as a kit. It is useful to know the parts; it saves lives when a surgeon knows what they are doing and where they are located. However, that doesn't mean it's all there is to the territory, or that the sum of the result is based on correcting the parts. It just doesn't work like that. A specialist surgeon will tell you it takes years of experience to learn the huge gap between the medical license and the power to transform the patient. Both are required. Excellence in (any) practice includes experience – it is rarely instant or accidental.

ARCHITECTURE

In the sixteenth and seventeenth centuries when the study of the human body was developing rapidly in the Western world, during the Renaissance period, architecture was another one of the metaphors used to understand the human body. The spine, for example, was referred to as a column. Cells were considered the 'building blocks' of the body, as if it was made of even smaller bits that were somehow stuck together into forms (like bricks in a building). In architecture, the fascia 'bound' certain things together (such as these different 'building block' forms) so the term fascia was used in the sense that it 'boarded up' specific areas and appeared to support or scaffold others together. The focus was to remove the fascia to see the parts properly – discarding the very fabric they reside in by cutting them out of it.

This so-called fascia was considered to be 'inert packaging' – another metaphor to explain the internal body. When anatomists were able to explore deeper into the body structures, fascia was revealed and scraped away, like a kind of packaging material (something like the fibreglass you might pack in your attic or loft, to insulate and fill out the spaces). It was 'binding things together' like it did in a building and 'packing them out' to fill in the gaps, as a builder might do in a construction. Fascia was recognized as a kind of 'connective tissue' but it was never assigned any sense of its own and only very rarely recognized as being *everywhere* in the body.

Fascia is a word taken from architecture. That is the rigid, hard matter kind of architecture we rely on for our buildings to stand up. It means 'binding' and refers to a kind of board that supports or holds things together like door frames and walls. It can act as a sheet to augment the way something in a building is integrated with its surrounding wall or frame or floor. A 'fascia board' is also considered to have a secondary (but essential) role in a building.

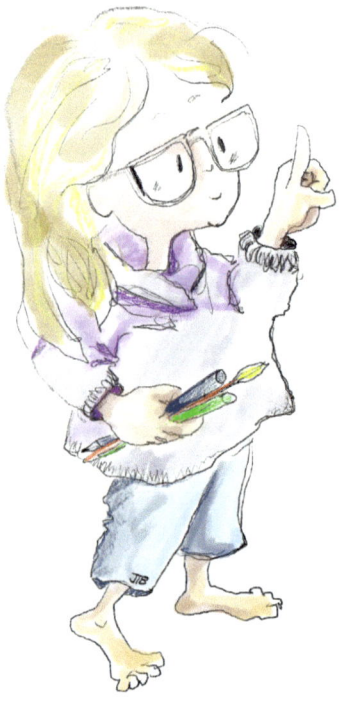

Figure 2

In the Renaissance period, architecture was revered as a skill and an art form, as it still is, that held great prowess at its best. Buildings that were constructed with grandeur in mind, from cathedrals and monuments to palaces, stately homes, and villages, represented the most extensive study. Since Vitruvius, the work of an architect included an understanding of the sacred, of geometry, of space containment and of construction, of how light was transmitted and sound organized in certain shapes.[2] It incorporated ancient wisdom as well as a deep knowledge of materials to meet the fashions of the era. Metaphorically, architecture reinforced the idea that something has to be constructed to make it whole, from parts and pieces. There's something even more difficult about the architecture metaphor, which matters a lot in understanding humans being.

THE MATTER WITH THE ARCHITECTURE METAPHOR

Everyone *does* have a kind of architecture, a living kind, however, it is formed very differently to a building due to one essential error that compounds the misuse of metaphors in early anatomical study. Buildings and construction are made of hard matter. You, me, they, all of us and every living thing in nature are *all* made of soft matter. There's harder soft matter and softer, soft matter, but it's all variations on the theme of soft matter, which is a different branch of physics to buildings and machines. It belongs in the realm of the cosmos, not the construction site.

The physics of hard matter and the physics of soft matter are very distinct. One is based on inert and stacked things like apartments and office blocks and tables and chairs. The other is based on rounded things that shape shift, often through self-motivated means. Every single living body is, basically, a rounded, self-motivated creature. We are made of cells, and they are *not* stacked like chairs, but *close-packed* together in tubes and pockets and pouches inside our living *soft matter architecture*. Cells are not, as John Sharkey puts it, 'glued together with spit and cement'.[3] They are bound naturally, by the tubes, pockets and pouches of what we call the fascial matrix, in a constant internal sea of shape-shifting 'fluxtability' (a word coined by Dr Karen Kirkness).[4] Living architecture is constantly changing *as a sign of life*, much like the cyclical changes in the cosmos, from moment to moment, with the movement of every breath

2   Vitruvius (c. 80 BCE–unknown) lived in the time of the Roman Emperor, Augustus. An architect and engineer, he was the first to provide written volumes on architecture. His work included the architecture of instruments, the study of human form and divine proportion as well as more classical aspects associated with the architecture of constructing buildings. He studied nature to understand form. Every design in nature, according to Vitruvius, included the three principles an architect must follow in anything created: *Firmitas, utilitas, venustas – durability (strength), usefulness, and beauty.*

3   See Release, Part 4.

4   See Recoil, Part 4.

of wind. They're not fixed like bricks any more than we (or our cells) are. They are in profound and invisible relationships with each other, unlike the parts of a machine or a house, that are essentially put together *after* the parts are obtained. We somehow put ourselves together, as if magically (and still somewhat mysteriously) arising from the wholeness at each stage of our self-development.

> *But cells are anything but inert, stackable bricks. The most successful efforts at creating living tissues or organs (for heart or liver transplants, for example) now involve taking a living piece of tissue or even a whole organ, digesting all the cells away to leave only the underlying biomolecular scaffold, and then repopulating the original scaffold with new human or animal cells. The scaffold provides the right structures and molecular cues to the newly transplanted cells so they can interact, gradually self-organizing into the emergent properties of the living physiology of the new organ. Neither 'engineering' nor 'building' is an accurate metaphor for this process. Rather, we are cultivating a healthy, complex ecosystem of cells within their molecular environments.*

(Neil Theise)[5]

We are held together with gooey ground substance, chemical bonds, and electro-magnetic fields throughout our tissues.[6] The detail at the interface of the cell membrane with surrounding cells is a miraculous geometry and the key to fasciategrity and bound water behaviour. All to be explored in the next book and covered in more detail in *Yoga, Fascia, Anatomy and Movement*.[7]

5   Theise, N. (2023) *Notes on Complexity: A Scientific Theory of Connection, Consciousness, and Being*. New York, NY: Spiegel & Grau.

6   Ho, M.-W. (2017) 'Water the Means, Medium and Message of Life.' In Ho, M.-W. (ed.) *Meaning of Life and the Universe: Transforming*. World Scientific Publishing Co. Pte. Ltd, London, UK and Ho, M. W. and Knight, D. (1998) 'The acupuncture system and the liquid crystalline collagen fibers of the connective tissues.' *American Journal of Chinese Medicine* 26, 251–263.

7   Avison, J. (2021) *Yoga, Fascia, Anatomy and Movement*. Edinburgh: Handspring Publishing.

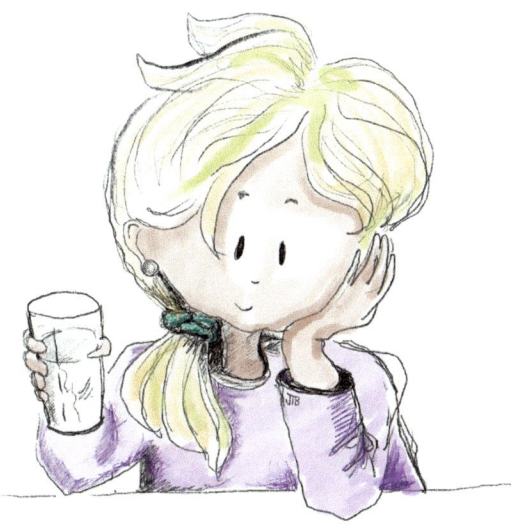

Figure 3

This era, like that of the founding fathers of modern science, is also a culture of innovation. Theirs was the Industrial Revolution. This is the Energy and Technological Revolution. They thought the human body was mechanical because automation was just beginning to happen around them. They discovered levers, pulleys, cogs, counterweights, and wheels as their metaphors of understanding how things (essentially manmade things) could be made to move.

The new era recognizes that beings are essentially self-motivated. Yet the new language to describe that is elusive. Every one of us emerges from a physical experience of self-organization. That's what's true. The basis of that organic process cannot be reduced to its component parts. Namely because we begin whole. We remain whole as we form into particular aspects (within the whole). We, whole-and-complete, emerge as a whole body being and we remain that way within the living body of our mother and our planetary orbit.

Each one of us is more a part of a vibrational ecosystem that remains whole and complete as part of a larger whole ecosystem, all living together as a collective within the cosmic field. We are not separate from it. Every cell is like a cosmos, inside us as a part of a whole collective. We are like a cell in the collective in which we live. Machine metaphors have sanctioned a kind of 'separate self-sense' that seeks permission or confirmation of state, from outside of our inner sense. Yet inside our inner sense is the most marvellous system of resources and organiza-tions and networks within networks and potentials (like apps in a way) residing within each of us.

Our awareness can access the physical, emotional, mental, and subtle aspects of our beingness and recognize within itself what that trans-mits. The being and the body are never separate. If only we can find the language to incorporate our self-sense and self-esteem to restore that wholeness! We can grow and glow from the inside out!

THE AGREEMENT THAT DIVORCED THE BEING FROM THE BODY

This language, of machinery and hard matter physics, has shaped the perception upon which everyone learns movement and manual therapy to this day. It literally justified the notion that *living* beings and bodies can reasonably be considered separated, let alone mechanical. As Iain McGilchrist points out in the opening quote, '*Since what you find is a product of how you attend, this* [resorting to mechanics] *is a more or less pointless exercise in making sure that both parties* [scientists and philoso-phers] *sink to the bottom in the shortest possible time.*'

It is understandable that the mechanical metaphor arose in the sixteenth and seventeenth centuries, considering how it first came about. Alongside the reverence we developed for machines as saviour and symbol of our time, other historical developments were happening that compounded the divorce of body from being.

During the Renaissance period, it was mostly illegal to study deceased human bodies, in order to understand human anatomy and move-ment. (Barbary apes were used as they were considered to be enough like humans for the research of the day).[8] The value of learning human anatomy from human bodies was a profound breakthrough on behalf of humanity when it was permitted, in pursuit of progress and the highest ideals of healing people.

There were rare exceptions, however; dissecting human bod-ies (that were considered sacred) was forbidden since the time of

---

8   For the previous 1500 years, Galen's work based upon Barbary apes (on the basis that they had 'similar' structure to humans) was unquestioned.

Hippocrates.[9] It was not until the 1700s that René Descartes formally sought official permission from the Pope to dissect human cadaveric specimens (deceased bodies).[10] The Pope gave that sanction on a strict condition, or 'turf deal'.[11] The Church would retain jurisdiction over the soul, the spirit, the emotions, the mind – in other words, the being and all invisible aspects of beingness, while Science could preside over the body.

Bodies (dead bodies) were to be considered separate from the beings they inhabit – segregated from the awareness or consciousness that animates them in life. That rift is the legacy every body on earth inherited as the conclusions drawn were applied to the living. It became the basis of so-called Modern Science – it separated the 'me' from 'myself', the 'you' from 'yourself', the 'they' from 'themselves'. That fact, right there, is great, big, huge. On a gross level it separated the being from the body – on a micro level it gave authority to the kind of reductionist reasoning that many aspects of science embraced and still rely on.

Nothing really changed that underlying rift; indeed, it could be said to have deepened over the last 400 years as the metaphor became the basis of the methodology. Early anatomical drawings, such as those by Jan Wandelaar (who illustrated Bernard Albinus' beautiful and acclaimed anatomy dissections),[12] were considered frivolous for the inclusion of nature and spiritual references in the illustrations. Artistic creativity did not belong in anatomy science after the mid-eighteenth century. Even nature was excluded from the reference. The context of humans living in nature gradually disappeared from the content of anatomy until everyone forgot it was a metaphor.

That valuable sanction came at a high price. While it precedes many of the life-saving surgeries and treatments we rely on today (and the

9   von Staden, H. (1992) 'The discovery of the body: human dissection and its cultural contexts in ancient Greece.' *Yale Journal of Biology and Medicine* 65 (3), 223–41. Ancient physicians were inhibited from anatomical dissection of the human body, due to various religious and moral taboos of the time.

10   Pert, C. (1997) *Molecules of Emotion: The Science Behind Mind-Body Medicine*. Foreword by Deepak Chopra. New York: Scribner.

11   Ibid.

12   Bernard Siegfried Albinus (1697–1770), Professor of Medicine at the University of Leiden. Albinus authored *Tabulae Sceleti et Musculorum Corporis Humani* (*Plates [illustrations] of the Skeleton and Muscles of the Human Body*), first published in 1747 at his own expense. He worked with Jan Wandelaar (1690–1759), illustrator, and they devised a particular way of using hanging nets through which to see and draw anatomy more accurately, using cadaveric specimens.

surgeons that work and succeed in spite of it), it has also cost something. Ironically, in the Western World, the being was divorced from the body, under the very laws that allowed medical progress to save its life.

In truth, everyone self-organizes and self-develops. The fabric through which each being does that is currently called the fascia. The aspect of the fascia that focuses on motion is the 'myofascia' and it contains some truly magical resources for those willing to look inside and discover them for themselves.

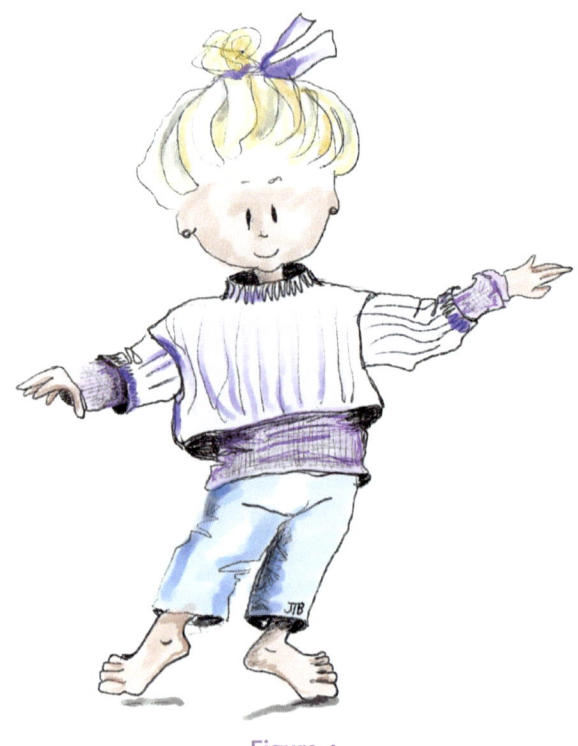

Figure 4

PRIVILEGE OF HISTORY

One of the privileges afforded by the turf deal described previously between René Descartes and the Pope, was the right of anatomists to dissect human bodies after a person had passed away. This replaced the study of Barbary apes to understand human bodies and motion, since they may resemble (but do not replicate) the primate form.

It really is a privilege when someone leaves their body to science for others to study it and learn more about anatomy for the benefit of mankind. It became the basis upon which anatomists learned *human* anatomy from *human* bodies. Clinical anatomists fulfil a unique role in Western Medical Sciences.[13] They teach medical doctors and surgeons to perform the high standards of technical procedures required in modern medicine and surgical techniques. Clinical anatomy could be described as a fine art as well as a science and it takes a great deal to learn. It is a privilege to work in the field, in every sense of the word, since practicing and making an error on a cadaveric specimen has very different consequences to making an error on a living body. It is the most privileged learning environment, particularly under expert guidance.

I have had that privilege, on many occasions, of studying in the anatomy laboratory, learning about dissection (which is not synonymous with clinical anatomy). The first time I did that, it felt more like being in a monastery than a mortuary. The atmosphere was sacred and the souls that had left their bodies to science, for whatever reason, sanctified the study that allowed each person present to appreciate, more deeply, the living bodies they worked with in practice. The donors, as they are called, had the generosity of spirit to facilitate the difference their donation could make to others who came after them. Working with clinical anatomist John Sharkey, Emeritus Associate Professor of Anatomy and Embryology Jaap van der Wal, and Professor Darrell Evans (when he was Associate Dean at Brighton and Sussex Medical School), were experiences that threw entirely new perspectives on teaching and learning about the fascial and myofascial matrix and movement. Each

---

13   In August 2019, clinical anatomist John Sharkey led a team of fascia experts presenting a Fascia Symposium to the Nineteenth Congress of the International Federation of Associations of Anatomists (IFAA) which is held every five years. In 2019 the Congress was held, for only the second time, in London, England. The IFAA Congress is a unique opportunity for medical professionals to share research and new developments in anatomy and anatomy research. Applications are peer-reviewed; presentations undergo rigorous scientific scrutiny, before being accepted for presentation. In the event, a presentation by John Sharkey, Dr Carla Stecco, Dr Vladimir Cheremensky, Dr Rafael De Caro, Dr Veronica Macchi, and Dr Andrea Porzionato was enthusiastically received by the large number of delegates at this prestigious event. In the same year, the professional journal of anatomists, *Clinical Anatomy*, produced a Special Issue journal (*Clinical Anatomy 32* (7), 896–902, October 2019) devoted entirely to the topic and science of fascia.

occasion in the laboratory was an absolute privilege. Among many wisdom shifts, learning to do a tissue sparing dissection with Jaap van der Wal turned everything I learned from the anatomy atlas inside out.[14] With that and the deep richness of his and Professor Evans's one-on-one guidance in embryology (a subject that could be studied forever with new revelations every day) I am sometimes lost in awe. Every time, all I can say, with my hand on my heart, is the human body is a wonderous incredible achievement. That refers to you dear reader, as I bow in deep respect for everything you have handled this lifetime.

It is important to emphasize that the distinction in knowledge between a dissector and a clinical anatomist is substantial.

The esteemed title of clinical anatomist is a well-earned distinction that comes with a wealth of knowledge and expertize. Anatomists dedicate themselves to mastering every intricate detail of the human body, guiding and mentoring aspiring medical students on their journey to becoming proficient doctors, dentists, and other specialists. Unlike a title under legal protection, there exists the potential for individuals with some familiarity with anatomical studies to refer to themselves as 'anatomists', implying a connection to laboratory experiences. However, it's important to note that these individuals [Author's note: much like myself] are engaged as more or less skilled dissectors within the laboratory environment. The designation of a clinical anatomist is granted after comprehensive years of rigorous study, grounded in strong ethical principles and practices leading to the award of a university degree. The clinical anatomists' level of expertize is highly regarded by surgeons of various specializations, as it ensures the precision and value of their skills in delivering the best possible care to patients. In the USA, for example, it remains possible to

14   van der Wal, J. 'The architecture of the collagenous connective tissue in the musculo-skeletal system – an often overlooked functional parameter as to proprioception in the locomotor system.' This article is published as supplement to a lecture at the Second International Fascia Research Congress, Amsterdam, 27–30 October 2009, with the title 'The architecture of connective tissue as a functional substrate for proprioception in the locomotor system.' It includes a revised version of part of van der Wal's doctoral thesis, submitted to the University of Maastricht in 1988, entitled *The Organization of the Substrate of Proprioception in the Elbow Region of the Rat.*

establish a private anatomy laboratory without the need for such an official title or extensive education, solely for the purpose of studying and dissecting the human body.

It is important to emphasize that the distinction in knowledge between a dissector and a clinical anatomist is substantial. The educational journey of a clinical anatomist encompasses a broad spectrum of insights and capabilities, unlike that of a mere dissector. This contrast arises from the fact that the clinical anatomist's learning encompasses a comprehensive understanding of various aspects, including and not limited to: anatomy (gross and regional anatomy, general anatomy, surface anatomy, systemic anatomy, clinical anatomy), embryology (e.g., including body organization, organogenesis, nervous system and special senses), histology (including cutting, staining, and mounting), human biomechanics, osteology, research methodologies, cadaver embalming and preservation techniques, sheet plastination, statistics and statistical analysis. In Scotland, for example, human identification can be taken as an additional model depending on the chosen specialty. There are also learning and teaching modules (i.e., becoming a tutor in anatomy) provided by studying to MSc level. Learning dissection does not necessarily include any of the above subjects. It enhances understanding of movement and manual therapies, under the guidance of a suitably qualified clinical anatomist. However, the distinction is a meaningful one.

THE MAGIC DUCK

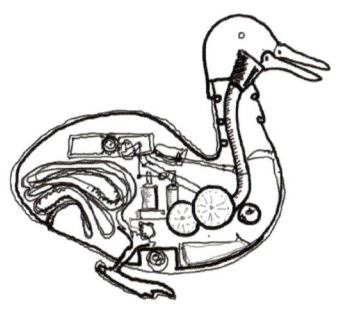

Figure 5

In 1738 (about a century after Descartes), a French artist and inventor named Jacques de Vaucanson invented some remarkable artefacts. For example, Vaucanson invented the lathe, which became very important in the Industrial Revolution. However, he is most famous for fabricating a mechanical duck that appeared to behave like a real one, when he was only 29 years old. The mechanical duck was made to quack, drink water, eat grain, and appear to digest and defecate the grain. Described as an 'automaton' it was a remarkable feat of invention and engineering, especially when you consider the date it was designed. It was quite literally 'beyond belief' in that era.

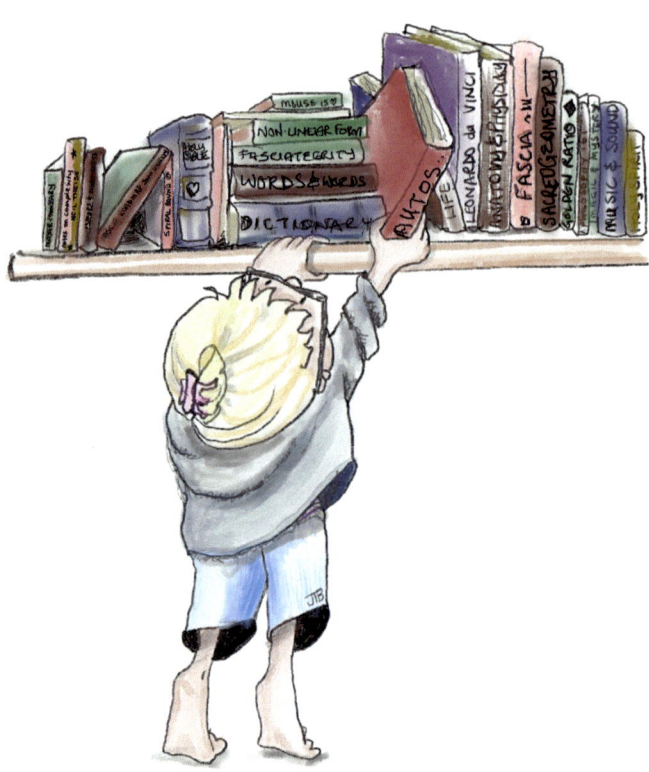

Figure 6

AUTOS: THE KEY WORD

The Latin word 'autos' means 'self'. So, an 'automaton' described a 'self-motivated' item; something we might now describe as a kind of robot. It didn't need a human hand to move it. Descartes had described humans as moving by a system of counterweights and wheels like 'any other automaton' – such as a clock (that ticked alone, once it was wound up). This was the theme of that era. The idea of being able to automate things was to progress by the creation of manmade artefacts. The 'creator' became the human who managed the feat. Regarding this duck-like mechanism in the context of the time or era it was invented in, helps to see how remarkable it was in the early eighteenth century.

To put Vaucanson's duck invention into context, the exceptional craftsmanship of this mechanical bird 'automaton' in 1738, was in an era of horse-drawn carriages and almost a century *earlier* than even the invention of the telegraph. The telegraph preceded the invention of the telephone (1876), the first car (1886) and the radio (1895). Electricity wasn't introduced to homes in England until the late 1800s, Victorian times. This remarkable duck, in the context of its time, wasn't necessarily thought of as a 'model' such that there was a distinction of 'mechanism'. It was as if, in his day, Vaucanson had mastered nature itself. The duck was designed by daylight and candlelight; there was no such thing as a light switch in 1738. In the context of its own era, it was 'magical and mystical' like nature itself, that appeared to have been *re-invented*.

At the time, it was as much of a deal as the idea of virtual reality today – to those that knew of it. The mechanized bird was so impressive (given the ability to 'mimic' a bird-like function and motion with its 4000 individual parts) that back in 1738, perhaps it was taken as something of a 'proof' that nature is based upon mechanical moving parts. This form of automation in a manmade object was beyond most people's comprehension. There was hardly any reference for it at all, as machines of any sort were not commonplace. Perhaps in the eighteenth century it implied that humans could somehow conquer nature. The duck had zero natural intelligence. It cannot and must not be considered 'real'. It only mimicked the appearance of a duck. It was like a duck. That didn't mean it was a duck. Humans in the eighteenth century were as spellbound then, as humans in the twenty-first century are intrigued by artificial intelligence (AI) now.

> Meanwhile, humans being form themselves embryonically: naturally, with no mechanics required and no parts installed. This clear and simple fact of life has somehow been forgotten in the scheme of things! It is intriguing to consider that the body can be studied as if the being isn't really part of the story – we somehow got lost in translation!

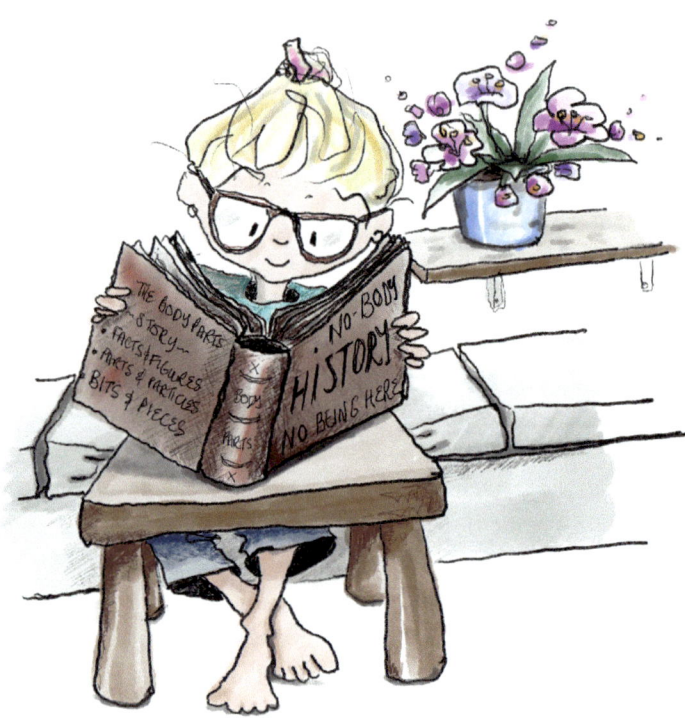

Figure 7

Back in the eighteenth and nineteenth centuries, the rift between beings and bodies grew; they were segregated from each other even more. The study of the mind (one of the invisible aspects of being human that came under the jurisdiction of the church in the West, in that turf deal) grew into the study of psychology which was separate from the study of physiology. Gradually, the healing arts became separate from the Medical Science and the metaphor deepened the rift. It was, in a way, a license to divide and conquer.

Through these two metaphors (of machines and hard matter architecture) and the terms of permission to do anatomical study from the Pope, human bodies were disconnected from the beings that animate them. And yet, it became even stranger: worse than the metaphor of machines and hard-matter architecture, is the definition of nature that deepens the segregation of humans from *their own* nature even more.

> The strange disconnect: the definition of the word 'nature' includes a variety of interpretations. Two of which are as follows:
>
> Oxford Languages: Nature is: 'the phenomena of the physical world collectively, including plants, animals, the landscape, and other features and products of the earth, as opposed to humans or human creations: "the breath-taking beauty of nature".[15]
>
> Collins: 'Nature is all the animals, plants, and other things in the world that are not made by people, and all the events and processes that are not caused by people.'
>
> nature. (noun) '1. the material world, esp. as surrounding humankind and existing independently of human activities 2. the natural world as it exists without human beings or civilization.'[16]
>
> The word 'nature' derives from the Latin word 'natura' which relates to nat – 'born' from the verb 'nasci'. Words like 'nascent' and 'neonate' have their origins in this root.

Since when is a human being anything other than a natural phenomenon, created by two other natural humans being? We are all humanmade, in the sense of being the *whole and complete result* of two other members of our species and part of nature's phenomenal brilliance. We are not *assembled* by anyone else; we do that ourselves.

No one else but beings self-organize themselves *as* the beings. Other

15   Oxford Languages (2024) https://www.oed.com/search/dictionary/?scope=Entries&q=nature

16   Collins Dictionary (2024) www.collinsdictionary.com/dictionary/english/nature

beings hold each being; nurture each being; maintain the environment for each being and provide the nourishment and waste management system for each being. We need each other. However, no one else put any beings' parts together at the outset. Every one began whole and complete and folded and enfolded and unfolded and refolded as one continuous piece of tissue that emerged at the right time, for each, *as each one*, whole and complete. No beings were ever (or ever will be) anything less than that. Whatever they look like, however they express themselves, whatever the fashion of the day and the local judgements about what is fashionable – *every one* beautifully *animates* (in motion) their nature in their own unique way. Moreover, they do it from the inside out.

The fact is that every one (like all living things) is an example of nature's emergent properties; self-organizing and self-aware; in their time, in motion, unlike houses and castles and office blocks that are static. Manmade architectures are made of many parts and materials and separate systems, put together after the parts have been ordered in bulk and systematically organized and shaped (by man) into manmade artefacts and assembled. We pray they are designed to withstand nature's unpredictability (such as earthquakes or high winds). Whether assembled by men or machines (that men designed) they qualify as 'something other than nature'. Humans being do not qualify for that label of 'other than nature'. That is nonsense.

Human beings are disqualified from any such assumptions. Humans are made of one continuous piece of tissue that they self-organize into forms that *form into their parts*, out of one tiny bubble the size of a pencil dot! Just as every acorn that grows into an oak tree begins considerably smaller in all dimensions, without bolting on any branches or inserting sap, or hanging leaves along the twigs or learning the skilled artisan craftsmanship of becoming a tree. The acorn never even learns to spell 'acorn' or 'oak tree' yet it becomes both, in time, all by itself with the help of the earth and elements. It is whole and complete at every stage of acorn, sapling, and oak. Humans begin whole and complete and remain that way all their lives. They are whole and complete at every stage from conception, embryo, fetus, neonate, child, adolescent, adult, and elder. Like the trees, they are shapeshifting continuously and adapting to manage the earthly environment presiding on this planet in all its expressions. It is a process, a work in progress at every stage; however, it is unique work all the time, everywhere by every one.[17]

There is actually little or no comparison between the fascia boards of a house with the fascia matrix of a body. No one arose from the parts being put together. The only thing they have loosely in common is a role of *binding*. Houses are inert; humans being are anything but inert (unless they're dead)! Movement is the sign of life. Myofascial magic depends on it – and so does the science and experience behind it. It can be called an expression of the 'New Science of Body Architecture'[18] – however, there first has to be an acceptance of the basic laws of soft matter and living, non-linear biologic forms (which are not mechanical) and the very unique way their architecture is animated.

The magic ingredient comes from understanding the 'how' of self-organization. Humans are made of soft matter, not hard matter, however spellbinding the historical explanations are. It already *is* human nature to be round, surrounded, and organized as a biomotionally intelligent, adaptable soft-matter form, mostly grounded in gravity. Within that is a range of soft-soft matter and harder-soft matter – however, it is all always (when healthy) metabolizing and adapting form, to serve each individual it belongs to *in the round*. Everyone is made of soft matter. Everyone is governed by its laws, in spite of what they might like to think!

Soft matter architecture's structural integrity is based entirely in containments of spheres and variations on a spherical, lattice-like, tubular theme. Humans begin whole and complete, *in the round*. Everyone *always* self-organizes the parts into being, from within that rounded wholeness, inside the containing skin. It is a whole other geometry to squares and cubes and rectangles stuck together like bricks. It includes all of the shapes in the spectrum; however, it isn't about stacked blocks. It's all about triangulation and the geometry of spheres and the spaces between them and how they close-pack, rather than stack (it's a different kind of relationship and it holds the secret of our structural integrity). They are pressed (compressing) together by their surrounding skins and they push apart (tensioning) in response.

---

17 Sharkey, J. (2023) 'Fascia as a process.' https://myofascialmagic.com/post/fascia-as-a-process
18 See Chapter 3: From Anatomy to Architecture, in Avison, *Yoga, Fascia, Anatomy and Movement*, 2E.

That can be said the other way around, too. (See Part 3, The Magic.) That dance, that living reciprocal process of life-force containing (pushing out – centrifugally) and responding (pushing in – centripetally) in 360 degrees of omni-directional transmission, is our living pulse. Always. In. The. Round. I know – go figure!

Each being is the architect that self-wove the architecture to express themselves as the architect.

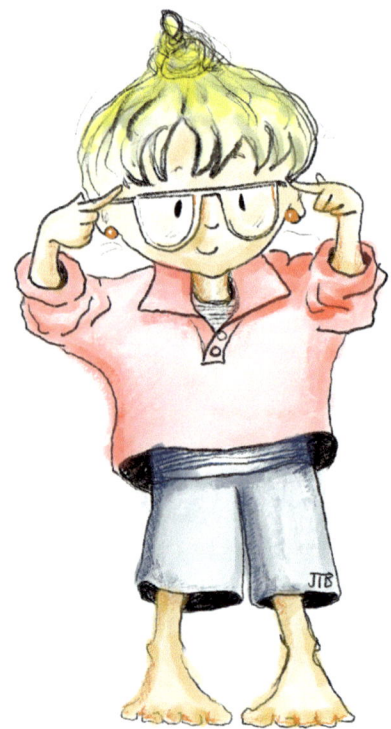

Figure 8

The foundation (of soft matter) requires some new metaphors to carry every one of us humans being into an era of connectivity and collective awareness. It is essential to join the dots of our self-initiated progress. That is from egg to elder and from era to era.

THE INTERNET AND THE INTERNALNET
– A DIFFERENT METAPHOR

We are living organisms, and our natural operating system is not based on mechanical parts or machines. New metaphors are needed to begin understanding how the being and the body are already working, if there is nothing mechanical or linear about us.

We are structured much more like the invisible 'worldwide webs' of the internet, the smart screen interfaces and the multidimensional subtleties of our personalized apps; things we understand in this modern era of networks. Our physical awareness is actually based on something we didn't have the means to examine or describe until this, the twenty-first century. Ironically, it is the technological revolution of this era that is drawing attention to a new level of metaphor! (Several, in fact).

Human beings of the twenty-first century speak a different language to the founding fathers. We have words like 'networks' and 'optimization', 'service provider', and 'UX' for user experience.

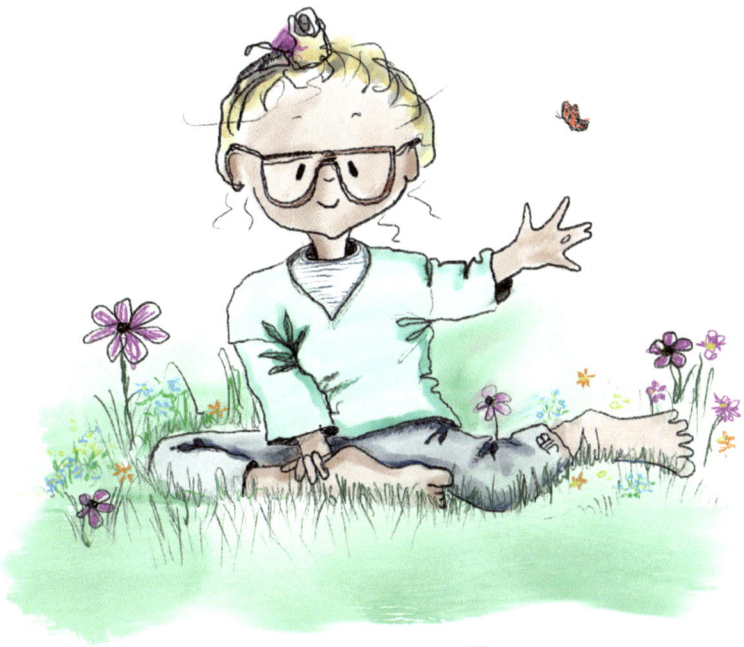

Figure 9

Let it be said that computers and the internet are not an ideal metaphor for the human body either, although they certainly provide an upgrade on the industrial machine. The following words (among others) were removed from the children's dictionary to make way for new words that are called for by use of computers and the internet.[19] Deleted words were: acorn, bluebell, buttercup, dandelion, fern, kingfisher, lark, mistletoe, nectar, otter, willow. New words that have been included in the dictionary are: broadband, cut and paste, analogue. Perhaps we have to be as careful about ignoring nature now as when Vaucanson thought he had mastered it. Who knows?

Every one has a unique way of relating to their own unbelievably sophisticated smart phones/tablets/computers. There is a worldwide reliance, knowingly or not, on 'sounds and haptics'. It is one of the features under 'general' in a mobile phone's 'systems' section. It is inside the mysterious (for most of us) inner workings of a computer's preferences.

It turns out that the new science of body architecture explains the long-known (if underestimated) matrix of the human connective tissue system (that tends to be included in the term 'the fascia'). This system effectively represents the (soft-matter) material of every micromillimetre of the entire body from ground to crown. It is this that makes a new sense of living beings' essential wholeness. It makes the spiritual notion of interconnectedness literal and true at the most basic physical level. It starts with the individual. It is already a collective. It is already a member of the collective. Physically, emotionally, mentally, and spiritually – consciously or not!

Inside a smartphone (for example) under Settings> General> is something called Sounds and Haptics. Haptics refer to the 'sensory feedback' of the screen interface in response to touch. What that means is that when someone taps, double taps, presses, swipes and

---

19   In a discussion in *The Guardian* newspaper (Tuesday, 13 January 2015) reported by Alison Flood.

so on, the phone can appear to respond to subtle differences in the type of touch. Martin Grunwald is a scientist whose research can be found in his book *Human Haptic Perception*.[20] This is the body-wide internal network of the fascia matrix,which is capable of responding in the most subtle ways to variations in touch/motion of the human body. More on that in Mystery and Magic in Parts 2 and 3.

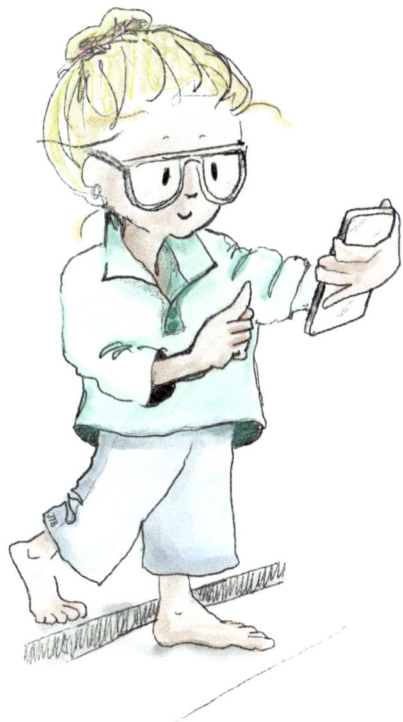

Figure 10

The fascial matrix, within which is the myofascial matrix, is a profoundly intelligent, internal sensing system that communicates and interfaces everything within everyone, with everything else – inside and around everybody. That is cell-to-cell communication – organ to organ, shape to shape, inner to outer – it is so essential and relentless, *on every scale*

20   Grunwald, M. (2008) *Human Haptic Perception: Basics and Applications*. Basel: Birkhäuser Verlag.

that it is hidden in the obvious everyday life of a living body as part of what is taken for granted in the experience of being alive. Every little thing any one of us does, every gesture, is part of the responsiveness of this internal intelligence network (much as a smart phone is part of our everyday lives). It *resonates* and creates a *resonance field.* This is not new knowledge, however, we have yet to find a new context to fully appreciate it.

Imagine a smart phone, a tablet, or a touch screen computer for a moment. It may even be how this book is displaying. It is a piece of hardware that has been installed with all sorts of software onto it – to make it work for the person using it. That person has personalized the software so it serves their purpose. Every touch, swipe, stroke, and tap, animates the lights and sounds or colours and effects that 'bring it to life' for as long as it has the battery charge, to display (and present the apps for them) and respond to that person's every move. All sorts of things can go wrong, and all sorts of things can go right, and every day is unique in the life of a person and their 'mobile device(s)'. All of us communicate with each other through the ether, via invisible signals and frequencies that are harnessed by the software interfaces each user personalizes. That software is animated by switching it on and relying on it to communicate back. It communicates back through sound and light (pictures and noises). It's called 'feedback'. It is the interface between the user and their connections around the world. It relies on bandwidth and internet providers and so on.

Think about that for a moment. Think how deeply connected it makes everyone. Regardless of the rights and wrongs of the ways the programmes are used, or the judgements of different media centres and apps, there is an exceptional amount of connection and interconnection and relationship between the users. Conversations take place at the speed of light and sound everywhere in the world, every day. *That very connectedness makes more sense of the human fascial matrix, than a mechanical vehicle.* Our globalized technology describes (more closely than in comparison with a machine or a train) the incalculable sensory awareness that every body relies on *anyway*, from moment to moment. Their survival and well-being rely on this internal communication system *whether they know it or not.* That internal communication system relies on sound and light. It is conducted at the respective speeds and it actually counts on them for its internal well-being. It is the inner world of human haptic perception. We have even adopted the term 'bandwidth' to describe our ability to handle things. 'I don't have the emotional band-width to take all this in' is a perfect expression of how beings-in-bodies reveal at some level their *biomotional intelligence.*

Human beings have unprecedented access to internal information and instinctive and intuitive sentience. Beings already are unbelievably complex integrated embodied systems – as responsive and exquisitely detailed as anything that they could invent. They never were biomechan-ical. It's so much worse than the wrong metaphor. It's reduced our innate and subtle intuitive range of abilities to those of a machine. It has limited medicine, movement, and manual therapy to mechanical methods and materials. The history doesn't need to overwhelm the mystery. Surely, they can enhance and inform each other.

What if human beings found out that the everyday interface of tech-nology communications was more like how they and the soft matter of the body work than the way it has been described for most of the last 400 years, at least in the West? What if everyone discovered that it was a more accurate metaphor in terms of its unbelievable sophistication – regardless of what each person understands about how it works! (Bear in mind here that no acorn has ever written a book about how to become an oak tree. It just becomes one – relying, like every tree, on a very sophisticated interface network throughout the forest floor, called the mycelium. The light, the chemistry, the geometry and the music of the winds is part of their story.)

What if everyone found out that their 'internalnet' naturally already knows much more than they think, if only they listened to it and spoke its language? What if human energy has been spent ignoring the internal mycelium of the organic, inner forest of our own matrix and 'earth'; the very ground substance we contain within and around the living primor-dial sea of our water-bound internal matrix? It is not a reasoning-mind entity based on data-driven quantifiable detail. It is a resonant field that each one of us contains, creates, and responds to, moment-by-moment.

The soul of man with all the streams of pure living water seems to dwell in the fascia of his body.

(Andrew Taylor Still (1828–1917), Physician and Father of Osteopathy)[21]

---

21   Still, A. T. (1899) 'The Fascia'. In *Philosophy of Osteopathy*. Kirksville, MO: Osteopathic Medicine Publisher.

MAKING SENSE OF THE HISTORY

The classical anatomy atlas

In the second half of the twentieth century, machines (such as cars, calculators and household objects like dishwashers and coffee makers) became commonplace. In just the last 100 years, road vehicles have become accessible to the majority and are no longer rare items for the elite few, and in recent decades it has become an issue to be without machines; at least a means of transport and a computer, a tablet, and/or a smartphone. Much of society, in many parts of the world, relies heavily on the advanced technology (to book a ticket, pay tax, park a car) that is now a part of everyday life in the twenty-first century. Technology has become the cultural way of life. It is changing language, it is changing habits, and it is changing metaphors as we navigate evermore technology-based systems to live and travel, literally and virtually. It is harder to avoid than to find.

It is rare to find a paper map inside anyone's car anymore, since a phone turns into a pocket satnav/GPS, guiding us, via the cosmos, in all directions.

Satellite Navigation wasn't available in these early jets! My father was a jet fighter pilot at 28, after the Second World War, a 'Top Gun' in his day. At 89 years old he flew a Meteor again. (This photoshopped image shows him at both ages!) Even the aerobatic loops were all skill and practice. He said it all came flooding back like second nature, even after 60 years! God bless him!

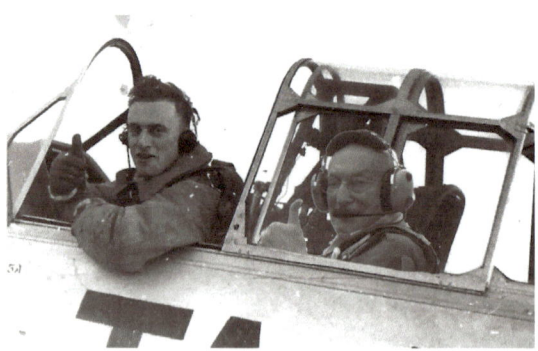

Figure 11

We don't even consider it marvellous that we can visit places in full 3D just at the touch of a map app. It is possible to learn, teach, communicate, and 'visit' (virtually if not literally) almost anywhere permission is granted to go – and our co-teachers and co-learners have the machines to receive the signals. We can't see those signals, we only see the results, yet we can now take for granted the ability to animate these invisible forces across continents. The point is, we can't separate the mechanics from the method. It arrives as a whole.

Nevertheless, anatomy (even the virtual study of it) is still based on the traditional atlas that shows the physical parts of the human body, revealed after clean dissection. (That usually means *after* the fascia has been removed in order to see the individual and separated parts). The territory of the human body is still analysed and based on the map. That is a picture of how a part *would look*, if the connective tissue in which it resides had been removed. Fascia was and is commonly referred to (in formal anatomical nomenclature) as 'a dissectible sheet or sheath' and more recently as 'a connective tissue matrix that surrounds and supports the body's muscles, organs, and other structures'.[22] It is mostly depicted as discrete points, or places in the body, showing little or no *continuity* with any other place elsewhere on the atlas.

Fascia is most certainly *not* assigned the impact of that continuity, or body-wide ubiquity, let alone the abilities of an internal satellite navigation system! It is not yet common knowledge that the fascia is considered the largest sensory system of the living body.[23] There is still a chasm between the current scientific research and the history such as we have inherited (described above).[24,25,26] That isn't to make it wrong – simply to point out that we are all part of an evolutionary developmental science,

---

22 Sharkey, J. and Flannigan, M. (2023) 'Towards a paramedical interdisciplinary definition of fascia supporting practitioners offering fascia-focused therapies.' (Part 1). *International Journal of Anatomy and Applied Physiology* 9, 1, 218–222.
23 Grunwald, M. *Human Haptic Perception: Basics and Applications*.
24 Schleip, R. and Jäger,H. (2012) 'Interoception: A New Correlate for Intricate Connections Between Fascial Receptors, Emotion and Self Recognition.' In Schleip, R., Findley, T. W., Chaitow, L. and Huijing, P. A. (eds) *Fascia: The Tensional Network of the Human Body*. Edinburgh: Churchill Livingstone/Elsevier.
25 Hoheisel, U., Taguchi, T. and Mense, S. (2012) 'Nociception: The Thoracolumbar Fascia as a Sensory Organ.' In Schleip, R., Findley, T. W., Chaitow, L. and Huijing, P. A. (eds) *Fascia: The Tensional Network of the Human Body*. Edinburgh: Churchill Livingstone/ Elsevier.
26 See Chapter 5 'Sensory Architecture' in Avison, *Yoga, Fascia, Anatomy and Movement* for more information, detail, and bibliography.

that may be learning to embrace and transcend and evolve from that historical basis of mechanical conclusions.

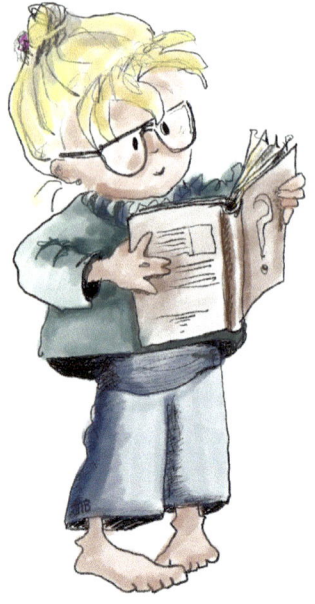

Figure 12

This was written by John Godman, an anatomist who worked 200 years ago and wrote about the fascia in a remarkable book called *Anatomical Investigations, comprising descriptions of various Fasciae of the Human Body* (1824). He wrote:

> *The following investigations were begun without reference to any system, and without the slightest wish to support any pre-conceived opinions. The conclusions drawn were unavoidable, even at first inspection, and their correctness was more firmly established by every subsequent examination*

commenting that:

> *The novelty of these descriptions will, perhaps, be the greatest impediments to their general acceptance, for it has been very*

correctly remarked by an illustrious anatomist, Geoffroy Saint Hilaire, that there are many persons who become furious at the mere annunciation of new ideas – like him, however we shall wait patiently, convinced that time fixes everything in its place.

(John Godman (1794–1830))[27]

The big omission

The keystone of understanding the fascia is that it is continuous and connected everywhere in the body. Paradoxically (it might seem), it also distinguishes one part from another, with different kinds of wrappings – even though it is all one piece effectively. Did the founding fathers throw out the baby with the bathwater when they separated the parts from the whole in which they reside and from which they emerge?

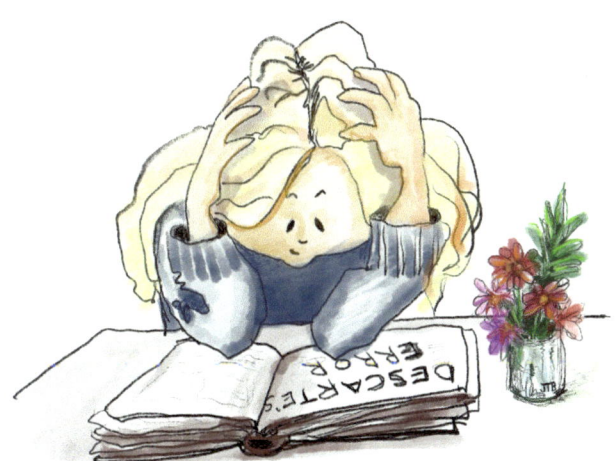

Figure 13

27   Godman, J. D. (1824) *Anatomical Investigations, Comprising Descriptions of Various Fasciae of the Human Body.* Philadelphia, PA: Carey and Lea. (http://www.biodiversitylibrary.org/item/89909#page/7/mode/1up) Digitized by the Internet Archive in 2010 with funding from Boston Library Consortium Member Library.

The growing understanding of fascia as a body-wide network on every scale, micro to macro, is changing the significance or the impact of that omission (of continuity and connection). The difficulty is that with the fascia in place, everything looks undistinguished. It is all there at once, within and around our complex internal networks, under the skin (which, according to Neil Theise, is an integral part of the fascia matrix). Unfortunately, the removal of it in order to distinguish the parts it wraps and connects, implies that those parts can exist without it. In a cadaver, they seem to. In a living body they can't – they arose from the fascia's folds in the first place. In life, those parts are intimately connected to each other. With very few exceptions (see later in this part), the separation of those parts was authorized by the predecessors that extrapolated how they might work when re-assembled.

The truth is the founding fathers were not able to find out the impact of disassembling them. We are still proverbial guinea pigs in that experiment! The maps or atlases were used to describe placenames with little or no reference for the continuity in which those places participate in the wholeness and continuity of the tissues they arise from. They had even less to do with the accommodation they located.

Nonetheless, the atlases provide essential guidelines. The point is that maps are not the same as territories. They provide landmarks and junctions which are super useful to navigate various ways around. They don't necessarily help with variables like the weather, or the shape and unpredictability of the landscape or the beings they accommodate!

Movement teachers work with the living, animated, multidimensional territory of the beings that offer their own feedback and change shape all the time; much like the weather changing the land, it can transform the experience of the territory on a given day. Each of us has a sensory inner network that somehow doesn't get fully explained by the sites on the map of the muscles, bones, nerves, vessels and organs that are labelled in the atlas. Knowing the names of the places and even memorizing the postcodes, doesn't inform anyone much about the accommodation that will be found there. It is a useful metaphor, carrying us across the divide with guide points, but knowing the names of the parts won't get you to moving well, especially if there is a notion that the metaphor (of a map) will explain that territory.

We have to join the dots on the map in real life with a different kind of awareness to anatomy train lines. We are, after all, non-linear biologic forms in all our roundness. The trains get us from separate bits to bands. Training can get us from bands to bodies.

Movement, as I said in the introduction, is not an intellectual process. It lives (only) in present time. It changes constantly as a sign of life, while the map remains static. Movement is an instinctive process that responds to the moment in the moment. The map is useful, it is a static guideline, a metaphorical tool, but it does not account for the being in motion with whom the movement teacher is working. They are not one and the same, however well the teacher can name the muscles, bones, and joints. The story of that being is told in the joined-up writing of their uniquely animated soma–soul beingness *at the time*, in 360 degrees of roundness. No lines, no separate parts, all being well – *a related being-body moving*.

The movement teacher may have a stunning and extensive repertoire of moves, but the ones they choose are crucial to the individual with whom they work at the time. Most movement teachers know this instinctively – for many, this is a relief and a confirmation for them. At first, it is very common to think that you need to know the map inside out, to begin to work with the territory. Knowing what the names of things are doesn't necessarily demonstrate understanding of how they work or what's going on here, now, where teaching takes place.

What is even more fascinating is that no one but the being with whom any movement teacher is working lives in that particular accommodation. None of us are separate from it or each other. The field we are in resonates relentlessly, subtly holding itself together *as itself*. The matrix is the communication medium via which movements are assimilated and forces are transmitted. That is inside the body-being and between them and the teacher. Why is it crucial to remember that?

The practice and the person

Well, it's essential to realize that everyone is translating movement their own way, into expressions that work for their form, depending entirely on what shape they are in. We tend, as movement teachers, to focus on the practice forms (the yoga postures or the Pilates repertoire or the action sequence, whatever the practice) – applying them to the bodies we are teaching – and even focus on 'muscle isolation' or specific exercises for 'joints' as if the map is all we need to organize their territory *intellectually* or *biomechanically*. The practitioner that hands a client a list of exercises is hopefully believing that they will make any sense to the patient, left alone to translate them into practice. Of course the map and the list are useful guides – however, neither provide an experience. A postcode does not inform anyone of the type of dwelling it locates.

Fascia is a body-wide sensory feedback system; it is a medium of exchange and communication – *through all the tissues our accommodation includes.* When our practice is focused entirely on 'a muscle' or repeatedly imposing a shape on the body – *are we serving ourselves?* If it is repeated too often, how does it differ from a repetitive strain injury? What difference are we making to our own patterns – or those of our clients? How do you optimize your given modality, posture sequence, repertoire to help make more sense for the unique being animating in front of you?

CLASSICAL ANATOMY

Classical anatomy is organized pedagogically as if bodies are mechanically constructed from parts and put together like a machine. The parts are taught as disembodied concepts, maps, codes, labels, and systems based on reductionist terms with no mention of spirit ever! *They can't live without it!* Yet the teaching is founded in this 'reductionism' as if it sanctions the study and method of reducing everything down to its component parts, systems, and concepts. We don't begin or end those studies with the caveat that anatomy is being broken down for learning purposes, to be put back together at the end. It is not distinguished as such.

This matters because it compounds a segregated, linear approach to practise. It makes it feasible to design classes based on parts and systems: Yoga for Metabolism, or Movement for Circulation or Polyvagal Tone. It gives out the idea that we can segregate the body into sections and systems and do the same with movement modalities to address the individual. No one arrives in class with their heart at home, brain at work, and body on the mat. It's a whole 'schtick' situation, where everything comes as one whole being!

Mechanical structure

The machine metaphor came into its own in terms of structure and function. Mostly it was considered that the bones were stacked upon each other, much like the floors of a house. The vertebrae, or spinal bones, were drawn as if they were locked vertically one upon the other, so the spine was considered to be a column. How do we lie down without falling apart? Architectural columns collapse on tilting! They rely on being stacked between the floor and ceiling of what they support, at 90 degrees to the ground. Humans do not. Humans can do cartwheels without their limbs or heads falling off. (These points matter, when analysing human structures. The failure to recognize them reinforces the wrong metaphor.)

The torso was depicted as stacked upon the pelvis, as if the legs carry it around as a passenger, with the head at the top, like the attic of a house. Despite the use of the term 'engine', Serge Gracovetsky (a nuclear physicist who turned his attention to the subject of spinal motion) dispelled this logic in a brilliant presentation at the first International Fascia Research Congress in 2009, and in his book and subsequent presentations and experiments, to demonstrate how the spine myofascially drives the legs, not the other way around.[28] The heart was (and still is) described as the body's 'engine', with theories of motion based on a system of pumps and pistons, like you might expect to be found in a car (in the modern era of pre-electric vehicles). The limbs are depicted as moving by various classes of levers and bending moments and the muscles are described as if they can contract and relax.

In this way, the body is usually referenced as 'biomechanical' and assigned functions on that basis. Even the most subtle 'somatosensory receptors' now recognized as replete within the fascia matrix have somehow acquired the term 'mechanoreceptors', which further validates the metaphor of a machine. The process is referred to as 'mechanotransduction' as if 'force transmission' itself is a mechanical process. It is progress in the sense of recognition of these subtle body-wide receptors, sensing movement within our form in all directions. It is a linguistic difficulty when the term 'mechano' is maintained to echo and reinforce the issues of mechanical metaphors. They behave more like antennae, subtle motion-detectors dancing within the tissues all the time. It can be more like describing the weather than the predictable data of a machine. Humans are not explained away by feedback such as would be expected

28   Serge Gracovetsky (1997) 'Linking the Spinal Engine with the Legs: A Theory of Human Gait.' In Vleeming, A., Mooney, V., Dorman, T., Snijders, C. and Stoeckert, R. (eds) *Movement, Stability and Low Back Pain – The Essential Role of the Pelvis*. Edinburgh: Churchill Livingstone.

from the instruments on the dashboard of a car. They may indicate certain information – however, they don't explain natural motion. (It is hardly a new idea to rail against reductionism!) Yet it continues in the very foundation of the metaphor upon which the study of human motion is based.

> We are not mechanical. Any movement teacher or dancer knows how much skill is required to do robotic dancing, it is learned, not innate! The body has to adapt to it, it is anything but natural – it has to be *imposed over* the natural way we move!

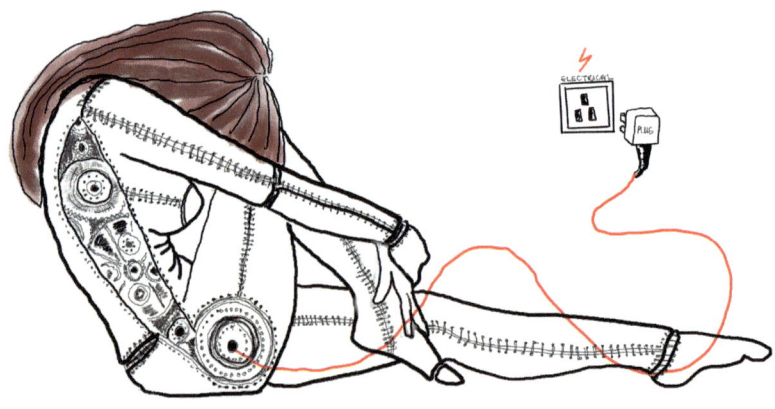

Figure 14

In classical anatomy, when we learn medicine, or manual or movement therapies for example, the musculo-skeletal system (our muscles and bones) form one of the primary systems to learn about for understanding the body in action. The roads and avenues of movement, the means of expressing physical potential and human performance, are most often measured by the efficiency of this system and how 'well' it functions. That is in terms of grades in performance or measuring criteria of abilities as data. Often muscles are 'trained in isolation' based on how they 'contract and relax' in order to function.

All those pathways to movement in the anatomy atlas are studied, while it provides the names of every area, or location, in the musculo-skeletal system, as it is traditionally called. That is the names of each muscle and the name of the attachments at each 'end' of every muscle to the nearest bone. They are the traditional 'parts' that form the so-called locomotor system. What if there are no origins and insertions, and muscles are not separate, but part of a body-wide biomotional continuum? What if those muscles are not what they've been reduced to in order to study them separately, *as if* they ever exist as such?

Separately (at the next level of training perhaps), the nervous system is added to the musculo-skeletal system. The lists of muscles show the 'origin and insertion and activating nerve' for each muscle. This reinforces the idea that each one acts as an independent unit and can be trained in isolation.

> *Because of the relative ease with which the nervous system can be studied, and because of its obvious importance, the brain has been studied with a vast array of analytical tools, and we know enough about it to fill many books and journals. However, one does not have to dig very deep into this literature to find that there are many unanswered questions. For example, the recent discovery that the connective tissue cells in the brain also form a communication system has returned the whole of neuroscience to the drawing board.*

> (James L. Oschman)[29]

The classical map of the nervous system generally resembles a telephone wiring system, and we learn input and output pathways of each nerve, and the general view of the central, peripheral, and autonomic nervous system circuits.

How do we integrate that to make sense in motion? It goes without question that they are intimately related systems – but what if that integration is completely transformed with the simple knowledge that muscles never relax, the fascia of the muscles (myofascia) and the nerves (neurofascia) is all sensory and responding faster than the nervous system and all designed under tension in order to spring load the original body structure? What if they are all so intimately related that there are no separate muscles, really? What if something more than a neuron instinctively animates our

29   Oschman, J. L. (2012) 'Fascia as a Body-Wide Communication System.' In Schleip, R., Findley, T. W., Chaitow, L. and Huijing, P. A. (eds) *Fascia: The Tensional Network of the Human Body*. Edinburgh: Churchill Livingstone.

movement? What if the study of reflexes and nature's built-in biomotional brilliance accounts for the subtle, intimate ability within every body that is uniquely expressed by every individual? Already. Anyway.

Let it be said again, muscles don't relax – ever. Muscles only contract. (See Release by John Sharkey in Part 4.) Their predisposition to contract is inhibited by the sensory nervous system. That means relaxation is an ability. It is a performance. It is even an achievement of an organized nervous system, which is made of the even more subtle communications of the sensory fascial matrix.[30,31] Humans are potentially as profoundly self-aware and self-organizing as it is possible to be. The mind of a being might not have any more knowledge of its capabilities than an acorn knows about its oak-tree-ness, but the oak tree potential is in there 24/7. It grows beautifully into itself anyway.

The first 20 minutes in a dissection laboratory, if preconceived notions are set aside, casts a new light on muscle attachments, the variety between human bodies and the variations in muscles from one side of the body to the other, let alone one body to another.

According to Oschman, *'a single-celled paramecium swims gracefully, avoids predators, finds food, mates, and has sex, all without a single synapse.'*[32] He quotes Sherrington in 1951, *'Of nerve there is no trace. But the cell framework, the cytoskeleton might serve.'*

This inherent reliance on structure, on the cell framework (what we will call the 'fasciategrity structure'), allows this organism a life-saving relationship with its environment. We already incorporate all that ability (or wisdom) within our own cell structure, and it is a body-wide intelligence that does not rely on levers or biomechanics. They don't exist in living bodies – however long they've been the chosen metaphor. At the very least, every muscle is invested in (and lives inside) a fascial matrix, so it is myofascia anyway, capable of neuromyofascial organization that relies on every other expression of the fascial matrix (blood vessels, bones, cartilage, lymph, and so on) to function. Nothing happens in isolation in the human body, so the idea that a muscle can be isolated in order to work on it becomes an even more mysterious premise after

30   Ingber, D. E. (1997) 'Integrins, Tensegrity, and Mechanotransduction.' *Gravitational and Space Biology Bulletin 10* (2), 49–55.

31   Langevin, H. M. (2006) 'Connective tissue: a body-wide signalling network?' *Medical Hypotheses 66* (6), 1074–1077.

32   Oschman, 'Fascia as a Body-Wide Communication System.'

investigation in the anatomy lab. (The anatomy lab being where the ubiquitous continuity is revealed, before it is cut up into parts with a scalpel.)

Hard matter architecture

The definition of a column is a stacked, compression structure in hard-matter architecture. In soft matter, there is no such thing. The human spine is an exquisite example of interrelated, woven tissues – organized under the laws of nature's most sacred geometry. It is designed to curve, twist, bend, fold, support, respond, rotate, restore and reverberate from the inside outward, with every move we make. It may form a tube of sorts, within a tube, within a tube (spinal cord within vertebral tube within a ligamentous tube), however, it never acts as an architectural column as if it was made of hard-matter materials. It is naturally curved and changing and designed in a very particular way to keep the torso pre-stiffened (in other words, the torso doesn't deflate; the spine and ribs keep it 'open' like an umbrella – see Part 3). It is designed to integrate variation.

The human body forms at such an extraordinary level of complexity that it is little wonder progress hasn't managed to replicate anything quite like it, mechanically. Apparently similar? Perhaps, but synonymous? No. Most animals have a spine that is carried, at least in part (think giraffe or ape, as distinct from horse or cat, for example), roughly parallel to the ground. That is *not* the definition of a column. It has been said that it resembles a 'column of ants' or a 'column of soldiers', but the implication is a 'straight line over the ground'. The language struggles to make sense of how the spine supports and contributes so much to the bodily structural integrity, while incorporating such variability and relying on being curved. Even in hard matter architecture, a 'spine parallel to the ground' would be described as a beam. Humans don't have those, either.

Everyone (trained in mechanical metaphors and hard matter principles) is left thinking that human bodies move via a system of first, second and third class levers, with stacked bones on top of each other and a functionality that relies on the 'mechanics of movement'. The notion of an 'upright inverted pendulum' to describe the spine is as out of place in human movement as the idea of 'bending moment' at the knee joint. It isn't a joint like the type you would find on the handle of a slot machine because it isn't 'jointed' in the same way. The tissue inside the leg, to permit motion, is simply (and very complexly) spiralled in complete dynamic continuity with a change of texture, rather than any pins. Moreover, the accurate definition of a lever is 'an open two-bar chain with a pin joint'. There are no open two-bar chains in the body, any more than it arrives in the world with pins to facilitate joint motion – *it is the wrong metaphor!*

The Greek philosopher, Aristotle, wrote a book called *De Motu Animalium*, in which the motion of animals is deeply embedded in the golden arts of the 'Trivium' and the 'Quadrivium'. The Trivium was the study of grammar, logic, and rhetoric. The Quadrivium was the study of arithmetic, astronomy, music, and geometry. (Leonardo da Vinci's Vitruvian Man incorporates much of this exquisite and mysterious ancient wisdom and knowledge). There is more depth on aspects of this in *Yoga, Fascia, Anatomy and Movement*.[33] A keynote here is that, to pick one example, Aristotle referred to joints in the human or animal body as 'resting points'. A man called Giovanni Alfonso Borelli (1608–1670) wrote a notebook of the same title, having drawn a dissected dog's leg and tried to work out the mathematics of its range of motion and described it as a lever, based on principles of leverage. The notes Borelli made suggest that it was a lever (dissected and separate from the dog's body, it would appear like an open two-bar chain, because the thigh was no longer attached to the torso), and it bent at the 'joints'. This is using terminology to describe what it 'looked like' were a human to attempt to build something similar, out of its component parts. Borelli's notes were published posthumously ('De Motu Animalium' means 'on the motion of animals') and he became known as the Father of Biomechanics. To this day, awards are given in his name, so there is huge investment in the terminology that, from basic engineering definitions, is inaccurate.

The definition of a lever is an 'open two-bar chain'. There are no 'chains' in the body open at two ends, there are no original pins, nothing moves in only one plane (as a lever does by

---

33 Avison, *Yoga, Fascia, Anatomy and Movement*.

definition – no one wants a slot machine lever behaving like a joystick), and regardless of imposing 'classes' to imply different characteristics of levers, it's simply *not* how we use the folds in our limbs. It's how we make a mechanical object *appear to do a similar thing*. Think, for example, of an angle poise lamp, to which we add springs, so that it can hold its shape. Human tissues are structurally organized with 'the springs' in place – much more complexly than levers explain. The human body is so much more advanced than these philosophers could fathom at the time – having broken it down to its component parts to imagine how they might be put back together again if, for example, Borelli was asked to do it.

Aristotle made sense of the *experience* of using the folds in our limbs, designed from the inside-out to *move*. The insides of our limbs and torso change *texture* to facilitate shape change. Discs between the vertebrae, cartilage, and ligaments between the bones form gliding fascial expressions to ensure appropriate hydration. Myofascial bonds (from ground to crown and all around) hold them in place, with skin surrounding all of that. There's not a lever in sight. It's the Emperor's New Clothes of the Body Mystery. Nature's forms follow the laws of geometry, just like all the other round things in the cosmos that Nature honours in *all natural expressions of her genius*. The same geometric rules apply to music and the movement of the spheres in the cosmos – which makes sense of the Quadrivium and invites us back to the resonance field of the great Greek philosophers who didn't reduce De Motu Animalium to the workings of a machine.

They honoured the workings of hu-man. In Sanskrit, the word 'hu' means 'divine'. The word 'man' or 'manna' is derived from 'divine (spiritual) sustenance'. It is fascinating that the very reverence that excluded human dissection since the time of Hippocrates was somehow lost in the pursuit of modern science. Looking back through the history we are left wondering if, besides their genius and wisdom, the predecessors threw out the baby with the bathwater, when they segregated the being from the body and dissected the connecting tissue (which no one forms without) and then reduced the rest of the body form into compo- nent parts (that it is never formed out of) and made up how *they* might put them together. No wonder we have lost our self-sense and our Wisdom Body awareness, as we discover we are already brilliant enough to create technology, as a collective.

The truth is, no one really has a 'musculo-skeletal system' if that implies it is all it takes to move. If the muscles and bones are the only noticeable players, then like the 'ugly sisters' in the Cinderella fairy tale, they only pretend to manage without her. We just think they can. No such system exists as such without the connecting sensory fascia holding it together, because the fascia formed first and each living human organized the muscles (myofascia), bones (osseofascia), systems (all vessels are made of fascia), organs (ditto, in fascial pockets), vessels, and so-called 'parts' from within the wholeness of their own fascia-based, soft-matter architecture. Even the in-between has a place and a role; namely the interstitium, which is the tissue of the in-between. It turns out that this is also everywhere – in a way it's the 'everywhere else' of the body and it unites everything with everything else. There is interstitium around and through every organ of the body, including the organs, the in-between 'virtual' spaces and also (not limited to) the muscles.[34]

Everything in every body is formed as one continuous piece of bio-organic origami.[35] Like the single sheet rule of origami, whereby it is made of 'one piece of paper', the living body of any being is made out of one continuous fabric, wrapping and enclosing at a variety of levels and scales. It is folded miraculously, magically, and mystically. Yet it serves us because of that. Daily. Diligently. The mystery being how long we have survived under a spell that suggests we are mechanical and formed as separate parts, before becoming whole.

Despite learning about the other parts and systems separately, none of them can exist separately. Ever. From dot-size egg to fully grown elder, every single body is whole, unique, and self-organizing in a continuous

---

34 Benias, P. C., Wells, R. G., Sackey-Aboagye, B., Klavan, H. *et al.* (2018) 'Structure and distribution of an unrecognized interstitium in human tissues.' *Scientific Reports 8*, 4947. David L. Carr-Locke and Neil D. Theise jointly supervized this work.

35 Origami (折り紙, Japanese pronunciation: [origami] or from ori meaning 'folding', and kami meaning 'paper' (kami changes to gami due to rendaku). It is the Japanese art of paper folding. There are three types of origami: 1. single sheet origami, 2. modular origami, where multiples of identical modules are pieced together, and 3. composite origami, where a model is made from two or more different pieces each folded in different ways.

continuum. Deep to superficial, ground to crown, inside to outside, and all the in-between. That's how it is.

No longer can it be argued that the fascia is anything less than a fabric enfolding everything on every scale of the body, in a way that can hold itself up (at its highest order of expression). Fascia is far from being the 'inert packaging' that has to be cut out and scraped away in order to show the important parts. It is now evident that cutting those parts out of the human fascia (or cutting the human fascia away from the parts) is removing the content from its own context of connection and continuity. A bag of watch parts, even with a manual, is useless at telling the time. It has to be organized, crafted, made whole.

Humans begin whole – even as unicellular beings.[36] Unlike a (hard-matter) watch, (soft-matter) living humans simply (and complexly) create the parts within the whole, stage by stage, within the body space, over time. John Sharkey refers to the fascia as the 'tissue of temporality'. It literally and symbolically (and metaphorically) tells the time in the body; accumulating every unique gesture it ever makes, in its own unique matrix. It responds in time and part of the magic this work delivers is enhancing the innate ability to respond well and adapt in a timely manner to what-ever we are moved to deal with. The fascia doesn't only work in linear time. Like nature, it incorporates cyclical time, and like the galaxy we live in, it also dances in cosmic time, responding to the resonance field in which we find ourselves. (See Part 2, The resonance effect.)

HISTORY IN THE MAKING

Twenty-first century anatomy – the dawning age of wholeness and continuity

In contemporary anatomy, particularly over the first two decades of the twenty-first century, things have shifted a lot compared to when classical anatomy was first studied on human bodies. There is new understanding emerging that is changing the explanations of how human beings each organize their bodies and their movements and their living architecture. There are new ways of scanning and seeing the body and new discoveries

---

36 Described by Jaap van der Wal while teaching at Kings College Anatomy Laboratory, London, UK, in June 2022.

taking place that challenge the classical explanations and bring everyone to understand that soft matter behaves very differently indeed to hard matter.

Humans are made of soft matter, right down to the nucleus of every cell within every one of the human bodies living. There are tens of trillions of them in each of us, so that's a lot of round things, all close-packed in particular ways, not stacked – or we would crumble when we lean over. That means we don't move, feel, grow, manage, or respond inside these living physical bodies *mechanically*. As I've already dared to assert, humans are not biomechanical at all, but biomotional in nature. The essence of being alive is that innate motion. The jostling and reverberating and hustle and bustle of cells in constant pulsating, living symphony stops as a signal that we are no longer living, at which point the body becomes static. At no time is it mechanical. At no time has human form, function, or motion happened without complete dependence on the entire fascia matrix within the body. That's not new. It's ancient knowledge. It's wisdom that might need to be recovered and restored, rather than re-invented.

Modern or contemporary anatomy didn't just discover the connective tissue matrix. It isn't new by any means. What is new is the recognition of its significance to movement and structure and sensory awareness, along with all the multiple roles connective tissue plays in the body. That is compared to what has been believed and assumed to this point. 'Fascia' is far more than a supportive, connecting scaffolding. It is currently referred to in a general way as the 'fascia', the 'connective tissue', the 'collagen', or the 'fascial' matrix. The myofascial matrix is contained within it – in a very particular way. Even the organs (viscera) are now being seen in the new light of the interstitium, the in-between continuum of so-called 'spaces' in the tissue.[37] This perspective changes everything that scholars have assumed, fundamentally shifting the metaphor that carries us towards understanding, by profoundly altering the definitions. For example, Alfred Pischinger, in the authorative text of 2007, offered a formal definition of 'one interconnected tensional network that adapts its fibre arrangement and density according to local tensional demands'.[38]

---

37   Cenaj, O., Allison, D. H. R., Imam, R., Zeck, B. *et al.* (2021) 'Evidence for continuity of interstitial spaces across tissue and organ boundaries in humans.' *Communications Biology 4*, 436.

38   Pischinger, A. (2007) *The Extracellular Matrix and Ground Regulation: Basis for a Holistic Biological Medicine.* Berkeley, CA: North Atlantic Press.

In 2009, Robert Schleip and Thomas Findley (at the second International Fascia Research Congress) suggested redefining the fascia as inclusive of all the fibrous soft tissues that form the organization of the body. According to James Oschman, 'their definition has the important feature of blurring the arbitrary demarcation lines between various components of the connective tissue.'[39] However, they don't include the bones or the dermis on the basis that 'fascia is continuous and bones are discontinuous; therefore bones cannot be classified as fascia.'[40]

Several key protagonists, particularly those with a deep understanding of embryology, contest this view. In part because the changes of expression (and chemistry and texture) of the body occur within the matrix. For example, in the embryo, the early anlage (plan) of the bones begins as cartilage. Through force transmission, these cartilaginous zones *become* bone. They do not begin separately from anything else in the body. According to Neil Theise, John Sharkey, and Jaap van der Wal (to mention three examples) both bone and skin (the dermis) have to be included in the connective tissue matrix. Indeed, even blood is considered to be a different kind of connective tissue that is studied under a different branch of biology. However, it is still a kind of connective tissue, so the difficulties of naming what is and isn't fascia remains an issue. What most researchers agree, however, is that the muscles are formed in fascia.

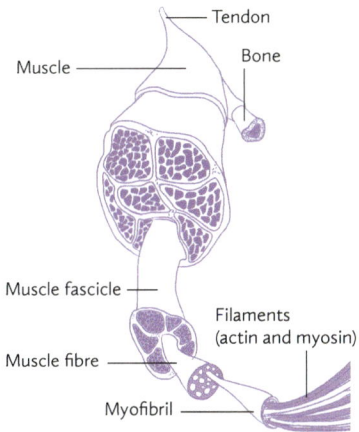

Figure 15 This is how a muscle is usually shown in an exploded diagram schematic on the physiology of muscles.

39   Oschman, 'Fascia as a Body-Wide Communication System'.
40   Private conversation with Robert Schleip in 2015.

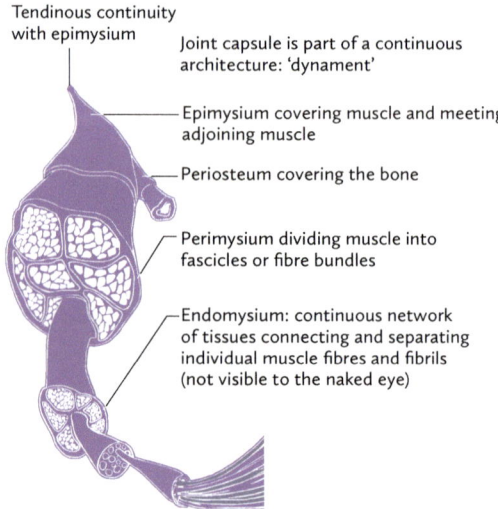

Tendinous continuity
with epimysium

Joint capsule is part of a continuous
architecture: 'dynament'

Epimysium covering muscle and meeting
adjoining muscle

Periosteum covering the bone

Perimysium dividing muscle into
fascicles or fibre bundles

Endomysium: continuous network
of tissues connecting and separating
individual muscle fibres and fibrils
(not visible to the naked eye)

Figure 16 The same drawing as shown in Figure 15 has been used to highlight the fascia of the inner (endomysium), intermediate (epimysium) and outer (perimysium) fascial sheaths.

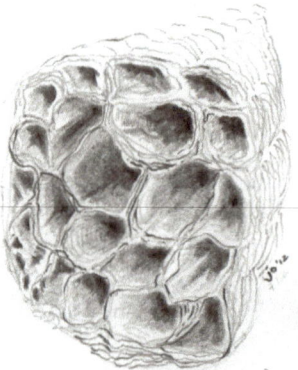

Figure 17 This drawing is taken from a photograph of an electromyographic image of the endomysium once the myofibrils have been removed. The endomysium is the deepest aspect and cannot be seen with the naked eye. The image shows the long hollow spaces where the myofibrils were and reveals the continuity of the architecture in which they reside. It has a slightly randomly shaped honeycomb structure and clearly acts as a part of the communication and coordination faculty of what is commonly called the 'musculo-skeletal system'. In the living body it is completely continuous with the epimysium, perimysium, loose connective tissue, and skin. There are no separate layers *in vivo*; they are an artefact of fixed cadaveric preservation. They may also be a language of convenience; however, they do not explain motion of living beings in bodies.

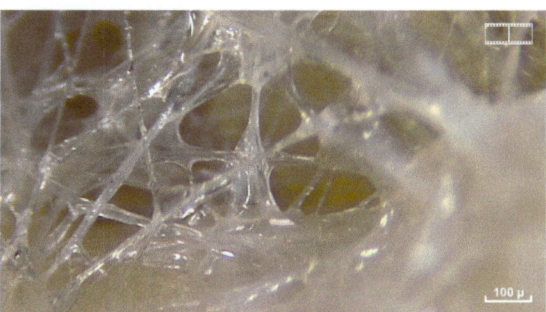

Figure 18 Essentially, 'fascia' refers to the architectural fibrillar network that holds us together, containing all the parts that make up the body. Whatever you call it, this living structural framework is continuous with internal and external connections, from bones to skin and everything in between.

From 978 1 80501 257 3 Architecture of Human Living Fascia.

Where does myofascia come into the picture? Myofascia is, effectively, the 'in-between' of the muscles, including their fibres, fibrils, and surrounding sleeves. To understand myofascia, looking at where it lives within the whole fascial matrix, or connective tissue of the soft-matter human body helps. Then, in many ways, it becomes really clear why it doesn't make sense to separate it.

Where does the word (myo) fascia come from?

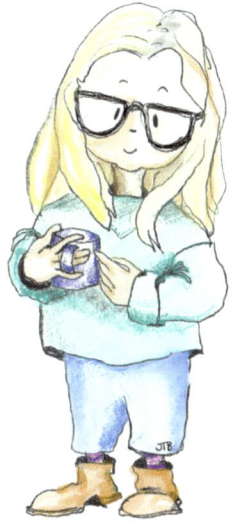

Figure 19

Historically 'myofascia' didn't really exist, in the sense that it wasn't considered to be a 'thing'. It is actually made up of a combination of two words put together.

'Myo' means 'muscle'. The word 'muscle' comes from 'musculus' – Latin for 'little mouse' and the plural: 'musculi'. (If you clench and release your fist, you will see the muscles in your forearm move 'like little mice' under the skin. That's where the name came from). 'Myo' is the prefix when 'muscle' is shortened or added to another word.

Fascia, in the most general use of the term, describes what Guimberteau calls the 'architectural fibrillar network' that is considered ubiquitous, meaning 'everywhere'. (Including vessels, organs, and the in-between of the 'interstitium' so named by Dr Neil Theise and Dr Rebecca Wells and colleagues.[41, 42]) Myofascia is one aspect of that 'everywhere fabric'. It is the connective tissue of the muscles and the muscle fibres that form them. These myofascial aspects are fundamental to our movement, however, the myofascia is not separate from all the other fascia of the body. It is one particular expression of it within the whole body. The one that each person animates, as themselves! (As only they can.)

Muscle protein resides inside fascial pockets that hold it in place, hold it together and give it any structure at all – not to mention its body-wide relationship with everything else. Most medical students consider fascia to 'wrap muscle', rather than learning how deeply it invests every part of every muscle, from the microscopic to the macroscopic. There is no muscle without it.

At the microscopic level, the fascia organizes the deep network in the fibrils of the muscles, within the fibres and the muscles themselves. It binds them to the fascia of the bones and in groups to each other. It also integrates the nervous system and the

---

41   P. C. Benias, R. G. Wells, B. Sackey, Aboagye *et. al* (2018) 'Structure and distribution of an unrecognized interstitium in human tissues.' *SciRep 8*, 4947.
42   See Chapter 7 'The Fascial Architexture', Avison, J. (2021) *Yoga Fascia Anatomy and Movement* (2nd edn.) Edinburgh: Handspring Publishing Ltd.

circulatory system within and around the muscles. It is the fabric of every vessel and form in the body. In fact, it is easier to think of the human body as 'One Heart, One Net, One Nerve, One Muscle'.[43] That 'one muscle' may be 'sealed down' in 600 to 1000 places, however, nothing is separated.

The truth is that everything is within its own ligamentous web and inside its own 'fabric enfoldings', forming sheaths and pockets and pouches that rarely resemble the iconic images in the anatomy atlases. It is all part of the organ system, but what has that to do with movement? Well, it has everything to do with movement because it is actually ALL connected. None of us can so much as sniff without moving the organs, let alone sneeze.

Every time anyone moves, all that doesn't move is also being organized. 'Organ-ized' is a key word and fascia is sometimes described as the 'organ of organization'.

Consider the example of an orange to imagine the different densities of the myofascia; connected to everything around and within it.

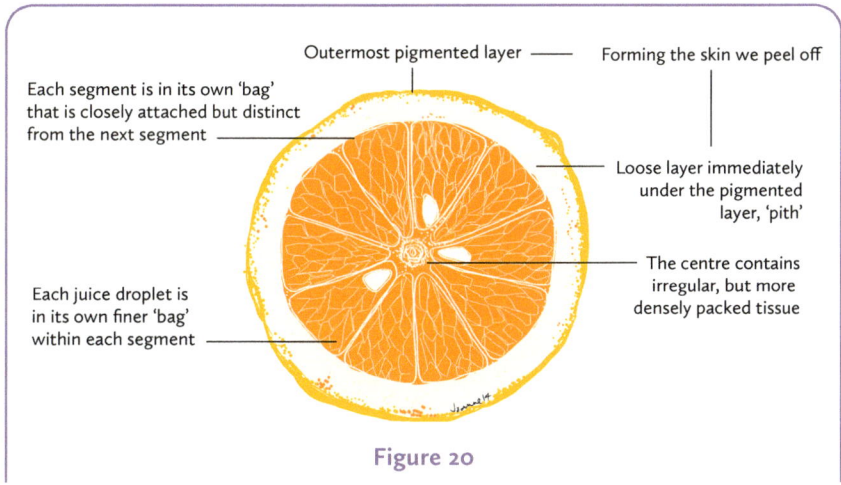

Outermost pigmented layer —— Forming the skin we peel off

Each segment is in its own 'bag' that is closely attached but distinct from the next segment ——

Loose layer immediately under the pigmented layer, 'pith'

The centre contains irregular, but more densely packed tissue

Each juice droplet is in its own finer 'bag' within each segment ——

Figure 20

43   Reference to course taught by John Sharkey and Joanne Avison at NLSSM in 2015.

Think of the outer skin as representing our outer skin, and the pith as the so-called 'superficial fascia'. Then that connects to the finer pith that weaves around each segment, which represents the 'deep fascia' and then the segment itself, would represent the myofascia, as if it was a 'segment' of muscle.

Within each orange segment is a much finer connective tissue holding each juice droplet in place, which represents the muscle fibres. You might also notice when you cut an orange in half, apart from a few droplets from the pressure of the knife, juice doesn't pour out just because it is cut open. If you hold a cut orange upside down, it doesn't leak if you don't squeeze it. The water of the orange juice is bound – just as the hydration fluids of our bodies are bound. You have to squeeze, compress, and twist (distort) the segments or droplets to release their juice. The connective tissue of the orange permits hydration on each scale; it is a finely tuned filtration system at every level. It behaves as a liquid crystal matrix, which is an aspect we will explore in depth in the next book in the series, on fasciategrity. For now, we can imagine easily that when the whole orange is dehydrated, we can't move it around very easily if we roll it. It loses its plumpness and shrinks and eventually twists all out of shape. Whereas when it is fresh and hydrated, we can roll it and has a certain suppleness, while retaining its structure (assuming we don't squish it too much!). This is, in part, due to the different densities and textures at each level of detail from the outer skin to the innermost core of pith at the centre. It is also due, in part, to the hydration of the droplets, the segments, and the in-between. That variety is a key to each of the 5Rs in our myofascial complex, as we will see later.

Fascia appears as a matrix – a fibrous matrix, to the human eye in, e.g., a dissection laboratory. However, in living tissue it is a completely integrated liquid crystalline matrix with a range of subtle expressions. This can be observed by the human eye in certain types of dissection only (such as Theil soft-fix). However, according to Mae-Wan Ho and D. Knight in their 1998 paper 'Liquid crystalline meridians':

Up to 70% of the proteins in the connective tissues consist of collagens that exhibit constant patterns of alignment, as characteristic of liquid crystals. Collagens have distinctive mechanical and dielectric properties that render them very sensitive to mechanical pressures, changes in pH, inorganic ions and electromagnetic fields.

(Mae-Wan Ho and D. Knight)[44]

This means fascia operates ubiquitously as a liquid crystal matrix, binding and organizing all living things as a whole.[45]

Cellulose to a plant, mycelium to the forest, fascia to the living form. It is distinguished by textures (as in the orange). I refer to it as our 'living architexture'. As a liquid crystal matrix, it can express itself in a spectrum of soft matter, from softer to harder within that definition and from more liquid toward more crystalline in nature. That is how soft-matter liquid crystals work. The tissue of our bodies relies on hydration, bound water, just like the tissue of the orange does. When we cut up a fruit it doesn't empty its juice. When we grind meat, it doesn't leak fluid. When we watch a child squish jelly (Jell-O) through their fingers it doesn't turn to the 98% water that it contains. The 2% protein powder used to make it keeps it bound so, although it turns into tiny, messy bits that the beloved toddler gets so much joy out of squishing and spreading all over their face, they all retain the structural integrity of jelly. That is the nature of a liquid crystal lattice, albeit a non-living one.

Contemporary anatomy inherited and still preserves these classical metaphors of linear, hard-matter architecture and machines from the great philosophers of four centuries ago, that hold us under their spell, even today. We have made incredible advances in technology that bring us to an era dominated by smart phones and computers the size of a postage stamp. We have the ability to watch movies, make movies, listen to any music, create it, do art, study science, buy and sell, learn and teach, laugh and cry together in real time and communicate across continents with a device the size of one hand or a folded envelope. We are even able to create 'virtual reality' possibilities due to our ability to understand

---

44   Ho, M. W. and Knight, D. (1998) 'Liquid crystaline meridians.' *American Journal of Chinese Medicine 26*, 251–263.
45   In Avison, *Yoga, Fascia, Anatomy and Movement*, this subject is explored in much greater detail with reference to Gerald Pollack's work on the fourth phase of water.

networks and harness the speed of light and sound and the means to constrain them.

However, in anatomy we still hold tight to the atlas as if it is the final word on all that we are made of. It isn't. It can't be. It is simply a map of the parts that are revealed by removing the very fabric within which they are contained and from which they were formed. As humans, that fabric includes the physical aspect of us, but it is not limited to it. The anima/animus that animates a being's every move sing through that tissue as a forum for their unique expression. It is as multidimensional as the satellite navigation system used (via the cosmos) to 'locate' a place or position on Earth. It could be said that it includes the metaphysical aspect, too. Where else can an individual spirit express itself in the physical world than through the physical medium each being is made of?

Is it possible that we transmit light and sound too? Not just metaphorically or spiritually or ideally, but literally as a presentation of our healthy tissue?

BIOMOTIONAL VS ARTIFICIAL INTELLIGENCE

Human beings are exquisitely designed to transmit light and sound, from the inside out.

That is physically, emotionally, mentally, and spiritually. I'd go one step further and say, 'Human beings are designed to transmit love, light and sound from the inside out' because everyone begins as an essentially heart-centred, emotional creature, most often organized with a bias toward compassion. That's as much a scientific statement about humans forming embryologically (heart first!) as it is a profound spiritual acknowledgement of the biomotional intelligence (BI), the human-in-motion awareness, the kindred spirit within. Every being on earth is a kindred spirit, in essence. We share the planet, whether or not we like each other. (Not all kindred spirits are so kind; however, we share much in common as humans being together!)

Moving into the era of artificial intelligence (AI), it is time to upgrade the understanding of how forming, moving, and being in the world, expressing ourselves through living bodies, takes something beyond mechanical function. It has become urgent, not just essential, to bring everyone home into the unique bodies where each being belongs, consciously.

The established story of the human body, in classical history (particularly in the West) is still based on this spell that relies on this wrong metaphor. It inherently (and hereditarily) spellbound learning to the notion that body and being are separate. That gave way to the idea that something outside of each being could direct it better than anything inside, that wasn't under the same jurisdiction anyway.

In her contribution to this book, Helen Eadie references Iain McGilchrist, who suggests that this mechanistic view is a left-brain means to understand things as if they are all separate, with no connection (see Part 4, Restore). Physiologically and psychologically, McGilchrist suggests that everything (from a left-brain point of view) is isolated, static and abstract, with no subtlety or nuance. It doesn't even move unless it is pushed to do so and relies on mechanistic explanation to order and organize disparity. Conversely, the right brain balances that view of separateness with a profound awareness of complexity and connectivity, evolving beauty and a kind of order out of being. There, nothing is disembodied or turned into something a machine could do.

Has the collective invented AI? Or is it just that culturally humans are beginning to discover and reveal the true genius and express the nature of nature from within itself/everyone? Is it possible that this collective is moving from a left-brain dominant reductionism, where even the 'self' is separated from the 'soma' to a new place? A place closer to translating the amazing subtlety of what humans already do, into the means to do it with more appreciation of the brilliance of the body's innate abilities? Can it be done with more joy and grace and soul awareness by finding out that the matrix inside of us is already as complex an interface as the screen on any mobile device we can hold in our hands? What if our ability to communicate intuitively is already capable of long-distance messaging and that the internet *replaces* an ability we have mostly forgotten how to use? One that exists within us and requires no outside sanction.

Is learning that the essential aspect of a human structure is a liquid crystal changing everything that explains the nature of humans and human nature? What if it resembles the design features of a silicon chip (which is essentially artificial quartz) in constant motion and memory, from dawn until dusk in every tiny thread of every single body? A liquid crystal lattice has a very different behaviour pattern from a machine, especially a living one. Would comments like 'the issue is in the tissue' in the therapeutic sense of a 'somato-emotional release' be a discovery, when what might be asked is 'where else is it going to go?'

The being is the emergent property, moment-to-moment and movement-to-movement of all of the parts that each being self-wove together as a whole.

Science has effectively (and unfortunately) reduced our movement to a complicated 'mechanical complex' of hard matter components. (Like parts of a car or a robot). We currently reduce the human body to those component parts, to describe it intellectually and in linear terms. We make up stories of how they function and interrelate based on those terms. Stories that science still cannot fully explain. However, the body itself (in spite of all that) has grown itself into form anyway, from a point of view so different to some classical science descriptions, that it's actually difficult to agree once the relationships of everything in the body begin to be more fully recognized and reveal themselves. Everyone self-organized from the 'materia biologica' that still self-organizes their world to this day. Everyone will continue to do the same throughout life, however they do that. It's theirs to do it with. They may not always be able to *control* it; however, they can optimize its responsiveness according to their needs and expressions and abilities. *They have a say in the matter of their form. We all do. The wisdom comes from within the form.*

The new science is in place to demonstrate this body-wide communication system, but the old language is an inadequate means to make sense of the new knowledge. We might already be better equipped to handle an internet world of AI technology than we think. Perhaps it has been able to become 'second nature' for the younger generation because it is, in a way, related to the primary nature of every living being. The speed of communication of our internal structure contains a certain mystery and a deep magic to its inherent organization. That isn't an 'airy fairy' idea – it is the foundation of folding and fascia as a living architecture – due to the way it forms, embryologically.

It explains why some movement modalities work for some people and not for others. It appreciates how every body has its own individual 'somatic pattern' or archetypes.

Part 2

THE MYSTERY

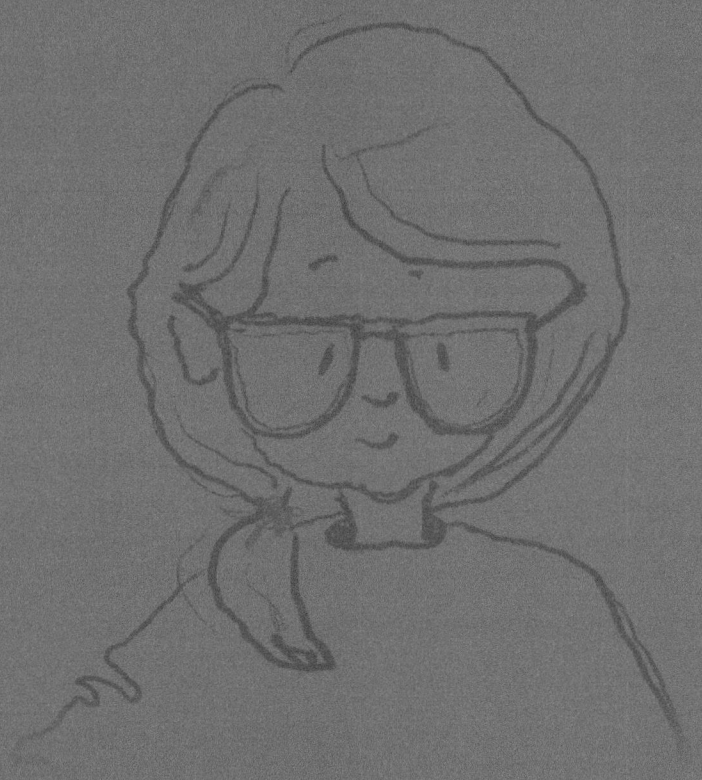

The complexity of all this rich abundance [microscopic life forms] has long resisted explanation. The origins of life remain deeply mysterious. What biological wonders might emerge next are beyond our knowing. If we were even to begin to fathom it all, a theory of complexity was necessary.

(Neil Theise)[1]

PRESENT AS MISSING

The human being is a wonderfully complex creature, living as it does on this planet all the various ways it can, with different environments, conditions, races, creeds, colours, cultures, and circumstances to manage and make sense of and adapt with. Between all the diverse questions asked and answers given, humans make the most marvellous mistakes and the most magnificent discoveries in this trial-and-error process of being alive.

Fascia is gradually being recognized as the largest (and most intricate and intelligent) sensory organ of the *entire* physical form of every living being. Regardless of the research and science behind that, stop and think about it for a moment. It means something so far beyond the assumptions of the founding fathers that it restores the mystery to the history that did its utmost to resolve how the body works – by breaking it down and separating it from the tissue of the architecture and systems and organs it sought to explain. Forgiving the ancestors and philosophers that preceded us for doing the best they could at the time is perhaps a part of the journey, as we, too, blunder our way back to making sense of the wholeness we were born AS. Every being alive maintains that wholeness, anyway, obviously. In spite of the history, it remains relentlessly mysterious. In some ways, that's what's so marvellous about it. You, me, they, all do the best any of us (can) know at the time and act accordingly. Is *anyone* supposed to know?

Mystery is needed. Imagine that the game of life itself is to discover the ability to transform that which is not, into that which is. (We

---

1   Theise, N. (2023) *Notes on Complexity: A Scientific Theory of Connection, Consciousness, and Being.* New York, NY: Spiegel & Grau.

might be the alchemists in training!²) Every being already transformed *themselves* from a unicellular being into a multicellular super-creature, capable of dancing and dreaming, in their imagination, if not their body. That's the fun (the fear, the fabulousness) of playing in Earth School; recreation for the time being.

Imagine the dreams and visions that inspire you – what if they are *supposed* to be beyond reach, so that the *process* of achieving them is the winning experience designed for everybody to teach and learn from? Imagine the fascia matrix of you is *in process anyway* and there is a way of rewarding it, replenishing it, renewing it, reassuring it, reciprocating its relentless guardianship of 'every breath you take, every move you make'³ as it watches out for each being it keeps alive, not knowing what will happen next. It also watches out and listens in to every being it relates to. Like it or not, the fascia is essentially a resonance field, mimicking and reciprocating the Universal Resonance Field each being is born into. It couldn't be less mechanical!

In the book *Job's Body*, Deane Juhan suggests the possibility that within every spiral of every thread of the fascial matrix is cerebrospinal fluid.⁴ If that's so (it certainly makes sense of some of the questions embryology raises), then this tissue matrix each person alive animates is the body-brain that the heart began to syncopate shortly after conception. It suggests that our awareness is indeed everywhere in us. Perhaps every part of us is listening for the next best thing. Our unique body language might be a dialect, or even a song, that each one seeks to sing and dance to, or at least play. Perhaps congruency of body and being lives in recognizing and voicing our own song, seeking harmony so we can compose songs to sing together. Who knows? Perhaps the best teachers simply facilitate their students finding their own voice. Once recognized that the tongue is *literally and physically* continuous with the heart (it is really one tissue!) it is possible to settle into knowing that seeking our own voice is seeking to speak from the heart. Embryology is a heart-centred sequence. Everyone did that already.

Perhaps it is part of consciousness that inspires humans to naturally

---

2   Meaning the ones transforming the symbolic 'lead of our wounds into the gold of our gifts' – Caroline Myss, Sacred Contracts workshop 2004, defining the alchemist archetype.

3   The Police (1983) Every breath you take [Song]. On *Synchronicity*. A&M Records.

4   Juhan, D. (1987) *Job's Body*. New York, NY: Station Hill Press.

seek to decode mystery and find simplicity to manage it. The founding fathers of the seventeenth century attempted to separate body and being and separate body into parts in order to understand it. That was a valiant attempt, based in the ethos of the time of 'divide and conquer'. Even the earliest embryology is described on the basis of cell division. Yet every cell multiplies into more whole cells.

Dividing and conquering the embryo didn't solve the mystery by breaking it down into components that didn't recognize themselves. The human being is the only model of the human being. I'll say that again the other way around. The only model of the human being is the human being. The huge difficulty in understanding it (in parts) is that there's an aspect somewhat like trying to look at our own eyeballs. There is an old Hindu proverb regarding the Three Great Mysteries, which are 'air to a bird, water to a fish, man to himself'. In other words, birds can't see air, fish can't see water, and being is almost impossible for humans to recognize. No one, after all, can get away from their beingness. It's always there. Wherever any one of us goes, we are somehow still there. Any one can only attempt to point there. However well-meaning each being's intentions, the journey is one of self-initiation, self-expression, and self-awareness. It sounds simple on paper – it might not be so easy to recognize or do.

'*Kindly let me help you or surely you will drown*' said the monkey to the fish, placing it safely in a tree. The monkey, no doubt full of good intentions, inadvertently murdered the fish. It didn't know what it didn't know. Welcome to the world of mystery every one of us inhabits!

The founding fathers of modern science intended to progress mankind, rather than cut it away from its own relationship with self-awareness and self. What is referred to as 'fascia' was (and likely still is) too deep of a mystery. It may take more than intellectual scientific data to unravel it. It may take restoring some of the ancient wisdom of the mystery and magic incorporated by everyone to *make sense* of this *sense making* organ of form. It is now known in peer-reviewed, gold standard, scientific research as the largest sensory organ of the human form. The recognition of that sends many sciences back to the drawing board. Not so much to *replace* the science with this new understanding of its significance, but to upgrade the questions that are asked in its name, in order to progress into the next level of self-awareness and human potential.

There were exceptional rewards for their historical discoveries – even if the context of nature being 'other than manmade' muddled mankind for a few hundred years. Mother Nature tends to be inclusive yet defining her can be elusive. Her repertoire of every species seems to 'try out' as many variations as possible. Every kind of moth and butterfly, tree and flower, and human being has its own unique expression. If only, if only, if only the most conscious species of the natural world could accept and respect that (prayer, not prose). Her wisdom is based in intelligence networks, be they the mycelium of the natural forest floor, the cellulose of a plant or the fascia of animal form, responding relentlessly to its environment *at the time*.

Mother Nature's hallmarks include variety and the exquisite experiences arising from the emergent properties of the moment. Every moment. Myofascial magic belongs to everyone, in the sense that feeding those intelligence networks within the body allow it to adapt for the experiences as they arrive, when they arrive. It's always unpredictable and variable. All we can do is optimize our readiness for whatever experience is lined up next. Predictable or (more usually) not. We can also enjoy the process and progress of that process, while we do.

Myofascial magic in action isn't so much a practice for someone to follow.[5] Myofascial magic in action provides various flavour profiles to add to and enrich the nourishing factors of any protocol. Whether it's fine dining or fast food, whatever the preference, myofascial magic in action seeks to make the best of *that choice*. It doesn't replace, it relishes and renews. It helps teachers to transform their own movement protocol into myofascial medicine, in the sense of a delicious resource that nourishes everything. It can rain or shine, this resource replenishes the network that (like the mycelium in the forest) feeds the forest floor and benefits all that live there, to better weather the weather – whatever it happens to be. It can be adapted and is adaptable to cultivate the kind of fruitful practice that feeds the body and the being it's serving. The overall intention of the years of study and practice behind it is to give everyone access to deliciousness in their own movement magic. That part remains a mystery, as some prefer focusing only on performance as if they are machines.

The next section of this book is devoted to the magic and then the last part to the five Rs of myofascial magic and putting it into action. They are designed as spices and flavours that a good chef uses to enhance

---

5   See http://myofascialmagic.com.

and create their own dishes. The intention is to create Master Chefs of movement teachers, while enhancing their subtle powers of intuition and instinctive abilities in movement. There is no 'one way' – any more than there is one species or colour or kind of bear or bird, moth or marigold, oak or antelope, crystal or current in sea or wind or electromagnetic field. No two beings are the same – they are not supposed to be. The methods and recipes in this book are tools and links to enable the thoughtful practitioner to transform what they do into something more resourced, more delicious, more valuable to themselves and those they serve. It includes some common sense, which has largely become uncommon sense – simply because it got lost in translation. To each practitioner, it is the unique wisdom (as a teacher, as one serving others) enhanced by that practice. It is one of the ingredients added to the intuitive and instinctive understanding of those whom each practitioner works with and for – along with the months, years, and decades of experience of each practitioner's own favoured movement modality.

In this section, the important aspect of the human fascial matrix that is a liquid crystal will be considered – if only to inspire the sense of mystery that each being relies upon. It isn't written like a scientific research paper, in terms of deep diving into crystal lattices and how they work. It calls to the common sense of joy and bliss in the sensory delight of moving around comfortably, whatever shape a person is in. It's the resource that allows performance to improve over time – rather than the protocol that suggests it is 'the answer' in its own right.

Human dissection (and access to a laboratory) is invariably a privilege. As a reverend, I have presided over funerals and experienced the intense pain of loss that people go through when a loved one passes away. Those two experiences (which are invariably unique and distinct) are very different in multiple ways. However, they share a particular common denominator.

The spirit, the soul, the anima/animus of the *being* they acknowledge (whatever the personal preference is to name it), is almost palpable in its absence. It lives in the awareness of the mourners, the hearts and minds of the living family and friends, reciting their prayers or holding their memories deep within them. It is invisible and mysterious. Their loved ones are present as missing.

Somehow, they are present in the very atmosphere among the people in the room. That spirit is not locked inside the coffin or under the cadaveric covers. That body is unmoving and without breath, it is what remains in the physical. The original being, the spirit through which they danced their body through their days in Earth School (literally or symbolically) is somehow still present in and among the beings around the body they left behind. It is beyond even the etheric realm; it is finer than sound and light, yet it can somehow be felt or, at the very least, respectfully and reverently appreciated. It is present as missing in the Unified Resonance Field, if it can be called that.

Beings who are still animating bodies, appreciating that spirit as they sanctify it, can respectfully honour it however it presented itself as a gift in their lives. All those lives are different for having had that experience. It is no longer physically in motion, however moved those present are by the memories or the donation.

What does this have to do with myofascial magic in action? Well, a great deal – because it is about the unquantifiable quality of a being that animates the body it occupies (or that occupies it), which is so palpably 'not there' after death. It has little to do with how many strokes per length of the pool that body could do, or how many beats per minute its heart rate pumped. All that is data. All that is (however useful) quantifiable information that is no longer very interesting once the data processing *changes* are over. Motion, change, relationships and connection denote life.

Static, unchanging separation of body and being denotes death. What remains fascinating, however, is the quality of the tissue, its texture and architecture. That tells a story of its own and it is writ large in the fascia and myofascia of its form, told in the language of shape and nuance of the network, stratified in the no-longer-living fabric of that no-longer-animated form, as long as it is preserved. It is something akin to the earth after a volcano has completed its eruptive journey. The stratifications appear (after the living turmoil and tumbling) as layers. They don't appear as such in motion – it is after stillness that static stratification occurs.

This has nothing to do with personal belief systems of life after death, or religious practices. What is being referred to here is the experience of the laboratory where the spirit, the anima/animus of the life force that motivated the body, is present as missing. It tells the *history* of all that preceded the moment of death. That story is engraved and embossed in every tissue fold of the cadaver. It may be very difficult to ascertain anything other than the most recent experiences (age, cause of death, etc). However, every scar and mark, every shape and fold, every minute detail inside and out, was shaped by (and shaping) the being that body animated, or the being animated by that body (whichever way around it is considered), since the time it was conceived. If only we spoke that particular language or read the story (like a sort of body braille) through touch, we might know what its contours and experiences could share. Every wrinkle, every strand, is where it finished telling that story and entered the realms of history. It would be something like reading the rings of a tree trunk to tell its age.

The mystery that emerges out of all of this, is what if we could tell something more than data about the *living* tree, just by looking at and touching it? This is not about playing 'Mystic Meg' waving parsley over a tree (or someone's head) and intuiting its/their future or claiming to heal it or raise it from the dead.

It is tapping intuitively into the intuitive resonance every single living thing emerges in and as. Every body also has access to it; a certain inner guidance that has a language of its own, if only we recognize the dialect. It is something other than databased measures. It is something that does not come from breaking it down into its component parts or reading the form detailing all the statistics. It lives in language like 'awareness', 'intuition', and 'instinct' that are so very difficult to define. It lives beyond words and explanations of the reasoning mind. It is often 'unreasonable'. It might be the Wisdom Body in each of us.

It comes more from appreciating the whole five-fold cycle of its life, from seed to tree to flower to the fruit that contains the seed. What if it could share with us the profound symbiotic resonance it shares with other living creatures on this planet? What if it has secrets that would deepen a relationship within us? Something even more tangible and repeatable than tree-hugging bliss. Something more like a profound communication system that offers medicine and magic within its mystery. You already know it can.

Anyone who lives in the wild, or keenly appreciates nature, anyone who has studied ancient civilizations or the history of modern medicine or herbal remedies, will know that this is the foundation of medicine. This profound ability to sense and resonate with living plants and 'know' their properties, understand nature's unique patterns and presentations, is where the modern medicine made today originated. Before industrialization, aspirin was found in tree bark – how did people know? Preparing it was a very different experience to our synthetic, manu-factured pills that arrive in a box at the drugstore. We might call that progress – and thank Heaven for the drugs and medicine (and surgery) that has saved the lives of my readers and the loved ones they live for. (Thank Heaven – big time!) The point here is to keep the reverence and restore the wisdom that *originally discovered* these remedies in their natural form, without science or databases to refer to. Think of the pro-gress that could be made with both aspects of intuition and intellectual understanding reunited for the highest good of all concerned! Can you imagine restoring the ancient wisdom with the modern technology, all based in nature's genius?

HIDDEN IN THE OBVIOUS

Fascia, in some ways, as the basis of human body architecture, is the page upon which each one of us writes the story of our life in present time, accumulating every stroke in the tissue matrix. It remains a mystery unless we tap into it and become willing participants in the sensory awareness of it.

Somewhere in your computer (if you know how to look for it or find it) there is a record of every keystroke you ever made throughout the time during which you used it. In a similar way, every micro-move a person has ever made is written in that body's tissue. The shape it is in now is the story of how it formed and forms and will continue to form and *transform* from conception to the last breath. It also *informs* (inside and out) constantly translating and transmitting forces *through itself.* It is never alone, and it is never without the dance of life forces within its bound-water matrix. It is always balancing a mysterious and complex pattern of geometry and biology as it accumulates and translates our experiences *through the forms it takes.* I call that the interface, with all its mystery and magic, of our biomotional intelligence. It's a resonance field that we are working with as conscious creatures who often don't know what to do. We find ourselves responding, nevertheless.

Every body on earth is shaping and shaped by the spirit that animates it. At the same time, it impacts the animation in a constant co-creative dance of the anima/animus *through* the form. That form is essentially made of fascia of one expression or another. The fascia could be described as the *interface* between the spirit of the being that animates the form – and the formation and shape that form is in. (We will deep dive on this in the next book in the series.) Not only does it make sense of the unique ways of expression everyone has *through their form* – but it literally is the *sensory interface* of that form, forming. This is not a discussion about the nervous system. It is more primitive, or primary, than that. This points to the fabric the nervous system itself is made of.

This refers to the original ability of every cell cytoskeleton to sense and respond to its own environment. When we multiply up from a uni-cellular to a multicellular being, every one of those cells maintains (or recycles) its biomotional intelligence; the sum of which is ours. It is in constant flux, responding to the inner and outer currents of our living experience.

John Sharkey teaches a gorgeous class about every cell of the human body, describing each one as a 'mini-me'. Imagine being made up of trillions of 'mini-mes' in a co-creative dance with trillions of helpful (hopefully) bacteria in symbiotic and constant motion as your sign of life. In health, that delicate microbiome relies on a subtle, environmental interface (cell-to-cell communication) just as we, as beings, work with each other to animate the same person-to-person communication. It is a remarkable scale-free system of resonance that we can find among all living things. It renders each one of us more of a collective ecosystem than a separate unit.

Each individual being (as a collective ecosystem, among other collective ecosystems) moves uniquely, balancing forces through their bodies as they move around. It is always a unique point in time, a unique space that is being occupied and a unique way of organizing it, within and without. That's what's true.

What is also true is that it never moves (bio)mechanically – it moves (bio)motionally or emotionally. It is basically energy in motion. This is not new information. What is shifting is the realization that it is *through* the physical tissues not separate from them. The human body moves because it wants to or desires something, or needs to move, or has a feeling that relates to a motion or responds to something (knowingly or not – it may be a reflex) and moves from or towards it. Energy-in-motion is *the* sign of life – it is what distinguishes each person *as living*. Not like a machine. Like a being. That being cannot be reduced to quantifiable data as if that answers everything. That body cannot sufficiently account *through databased information alone* for the living experience that body is accountable for. It is not a sufficient database to describe life *as a being experiences it*. Your computer has databases within it. However, your experience of using it requires software, hardware, and the person at the interface *to use it.* Any instrument requires a member of the orchestra to play it. Together they make magic.

A huge difficulty in the world is that many cultures base their achievements on productivity, goal-oriented ratings and standards, results organized around statistical data and 'winning' in terms of numbers and material accumulation. We still operate on a 'divide and conquer' theory. If that were all, then the world could be reduced to functioning parts and databases and it wouldn't be so painful when we encounter a lack of compassion or experience loss or shock. It wouldn't be so wonderful when two elite athletes achieve a goal together and share the gold medal as a mutual celebration. *Where does our sense of belonging to that wonder live in the body?*

What is true is that we experience these qualia as personal, subjective qualities. Moreover, our architecture is based in roundness, in 360 degrees of awareness and distinct qualities of roughness and smoothness, of fixed and flexible, of subtle and strong. We know balance by imbalance, pulling by pushing, reaching by resting, folding by unfolding, speed by stillness, and vice versa. Our sensory acuity gives us subtle distinctions between the hardness and softness of our soft matter movements. We are made of the most mysterious and magical soft matter tissue. It is living, gorgeous, messy, muddled, and grace-filled, not mechanical. Fascia holds the potential we seek. It carries grace, resident in the light and sound it distributes through each of our cells, each of the trillions of mini-mes we walk around with, making sense from moment to moment of our calling.

Four hundred years of academic scholarship based on levers and machines doesn't make any human being into a mechanical artefact. It simply breaks the pathway to their awareness down into its component parts, as if dividing and conquering were the best and only way forward. It is also inaccurate, so it dislocates our access to full congruency. We need that to *realize* our potential. Each and every body.

It has to be honoured so that we can belong to who we are – unique and exceptionally brilliant self-organizing creatures. Self-aware *and* manmade *and* of nature itself.

What if dividing and conquering were not the way forward and multiplying and connecting were more *natural* for progress? What if the original conceptus, the fertilized egg that began as you in a moment of 'unicellular being' didn't divide into daughter cells but *multiplied* into them? Growing in possibility and empowerment with every multiplication. In my world, when one becomes two, it's *multiplied up* not *divided down*. When a lit candle is used to light another one, neither emits half the light of the original flame. Together they shine twice as brightly. When a candle is lit and carried into a dark room – it is never consumed by the darkness. The light wins.

Pre-embryonic cellular multiplication results in more mini-mes. They are not divided down into separate bits; they all remain inside the containing membrane that surrounds them. They multiply. They fold into growing connections that form into the wholeness of each being, in all the multifaceted complexity of every body being.

What if the multidirectional and multidimensional awareness of this feeling, biomotionally intelligent architecture of being human – was designed to give us that experience with grace? What if it does exactly that? What if, the living human body, was nothing like a machine? What if it is, in fact, made of a liquid crystal matrix?

THE LIQUID CRYSTAL MATRIX

Which part of us is a liquid crystal matrix?

Answer: The fascia in the living form. The fascia with the muscle protein in it (myofascia). The fascia with the hydroxyapatite in it, forming osseous material (bone). The fascia with the cardiac muscle protein in it (myocardiofascia). The fascia with the neural cells or the fascia of the bloodstream (which is a different kind of connective tissue) or the fascia of the periosteum (that wraps and inserts into bone via Sharpey's fibres) or the fascia around every organ (pleura of the lungs, pericardium of the heart and so on). It lives as a highly specialized soft-tissue architectural form (organized by you, the architect) with different textures and ingredients that are variations on the theme of each aspect of the body, and each aspect of how each being self-organizes into form. Each architexture offers its own archetypal way of behaving.[6] The point is that

---

6   See Avison, *Yoga, Fascia, Anatomy and Movement*, Chapter 7: Fascial Architexture for more detail.

allowing that to be the case, promotes the facilitation of these subtle differences within our own bodies and between different people. We sense them anyway. We are moved by them – emotionally and mentally and metaphorically and literally.

Skin ligaments from the dermafascia attach through the superficial fascia (immediately under the skin) to the deep fascia around the myofascia (the perimysium). The deep fascia of the periosteum that wraps the bone tissues has 'Sharpey's fibres' that extend into the crystalized part of the bone (the outermost tube). Inside the bone it has the consistency of porridge, where the bone marrow resides. In between all the bones and skin are the different textures of fascia forming the muscles and the ligaments and viscera and holding the 'in between' in place. It all senses where it is in space through the physical communication with which the tissues connect.

Are we serving ourselves by *diagnosing* that sensing as if it is separate from moving well? In other words, can we afford to consider that the very living motion our tissue is in (that defines us as such) is communicated through the same tissue? What if the resource of myofascial magic afforded us the ability to recognize what we are sensing, intuitively and instinctively as a daily practice in self-development? What if it bypasses the analysing mind and simply shows up as the ability to move better? What if being able to move and be moved, is so similar that it forms *different resonance fields* of our growing self-awareness? Something inside us already? What if we don't have to learn it, nor can we cut it out – but rather it reveals itself when we resource it and tap into it *as a resource*?

STEREOTYPES AND ARCHETYPES

You are made of three things. Cells, connective tissues and the in between.

(Jaap van der Wal)[7]

The huge difficulty in science is the desire to establish the *stereotypical* nature of the forms. Part of the reductionist methodology, so deep to

7   van der Wal, J. (2016) Dundee University Anatomy Science Laboratory.

the way in which questions in science are answered, is the need to standardize and repeat something to 'prove it'. The beauty of the anatomy atlas (which serves brilliantly to a point) is the stereotyped landmarks that have assigned functions, fixations and formulas. All super useful – however, they don't account for all aspects of being in a human body (not a living one).

Stereo comes from the Greek word for 'solid', for a fixed thing. Archetype comes from the Greek 'archein' meaning 'governing form' and implying huge variation arising from that type. We all have archetypal patterns of behaviour. They change and style our gestures all the time. They are archetypal patterns of psychosomatic beings, souls in somas – beings in bodies.

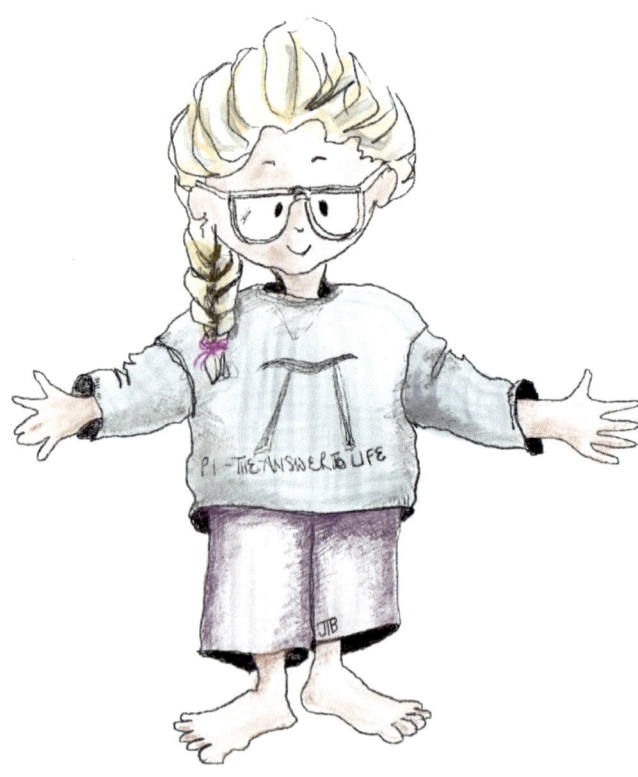

Figure 21

Everyone shares, for example, the type of tissue that is called 'myofascia' – yet yours and theirs and mine are not identical – they simply offer the same *governing form*. They are made up of a particular type of collagen and muscle protein. It is invariably expressed in unique ways. Everyone has a unique variation on the theme of somatic archetypes. Obviously. Everyone is unique – as we've said, it's what makes us all the same! (Equally valuable and variable in our differences.)

Fascia is archetypical, throughout the body, expressing a variety of *archetypal* forms. They include the muscular, bony, vesicular, neural, sensory, organic, visceral, circulatory, respiratory, interstitial, cellular, microbial, integumentary organs and tissues. In short, all the cells, the tissues, and the in between that Jaap van der Wal points out is 'everything each of us is made of'.

As much as reductionist scientific reasoning would enjoy stereotyping fascia into set terms of location, or specific function, or standard expression – it struggles through countless arguments because fascia is not a stereotypical feature of human architecture. It's archetypical at best and it seems to be requiring a certain bandwidth, a recognition of the being animating the body, to make sense of how it can best serve us to serve *its* integrity. We can't play 'divide and conquer' games within ourselves anymore – nor can we afford them on the scale of humanity. Surely, we have to find a theme of 'multiply and unite' to begin to make sense of Earth School.

We literally hold the memories of every keystroke of our lives, in the liquid crystal matrix that is our fascia. Much as every computer holds the memory of every keystroke of its existence, in the artificial quartz crystal 'chip' (aka silicon chip) of its memory quota. Just imagine the possibilities of human awareness once we recognize that everything about us has the facility to store memory *physically* as well as psychologically.

The fascia can literally bring the disparate and separate worlds of the body and the being, soma and soul, back together again. It calls us to honour the wisdom of the ancients, the subtle awareness of the intuition, the mystery and the magic of its (our) innate genius. It is no wonder that in the healing arts of various practices, the sense of 'release' of deep tissue, can (to quote Tom Myers) 'change the body about the mind'.[8] No

---

8   A popular phrase used by Tom Myers in his classroom, when I was both student and teaching assistant in the early 2000s.

doubt every experienced body worker has stories of how releasing pain can often be related to releasing a memory that was 'held' in place and resolved through treatment – as if they 'released' that knot or trigger point and 'the magic happened' (see Part 4, Release for more detail). These are not mad practitioners paying their clients to say nice things about them. These are repeated experiences that happen when they do.

THE RESONANCE EFFECT

One particular area of treatment where this feature is the foundation of the therapy is Frequency Specific Microcurrent (FSM). I've had the privilege of working directly with Dr Carolyn McMakin and using FSM as part of my own manual therapy practice. Dr McMakin (author of *The Resonance Effect*) has countless stories and scientific research, showing that tissue responds to subtle resonance.[9] Introducing the accurate resonance (in microcurrent – millionths of an amp – it's super subtle) of a physical tissue, through the skin, can literally transform its ability to release pain and reorganize its innate restorative capacities. In the event that the tissue can restore its optimum frequency (and FSM claims to offer multiple options where that is possible) it can demonstrably release the issues – often permanently. Without question, it can accelerate and amplify the self-healing systems the body demonstrates just by our species survival, and the basis of the forming or structural system that fasciategrity describes. *That pre-tensioned architecture might explain how the tissue has an original resonance field to return to.*

In practice, working with FSM requires a kind of trial-and-error process for the practitioner. Working together as a collective, the generosity of spirit among practitioners in sharing the variables *they* experience effectively upgrades everyone's 'database' as a collective resource. What each practitioner *does* with that database has to remain unique to them and the client in question. The therapy is based on accurately identifying the history, in an effort to (literally) tune in to the resonance of the issue and its impact on the tissue. It can become a super-power for many restorative benefits.

---

9   McMakin, C. and Oschman, J. (2017) *The Resonance Effect*. Berkeley, CA: North Atlantic Books.

THE UNKNOWN KNOWING

What if you could touch someone and that place produced an image of a memory, if only you could recognize the light or the sound frequency it reveals? Of course, that isn't an amazing idea – as anyone who has experienced a (true) medical intuitive knows, their inexplicable ways of body reading (or being sensing) seem to be outside the box of what 'should work'. What if that wasn't so amazing – it simply represents an ability that many have lost – rather than one that isn't available? What if, as Dr Caroline Myss will happily describe as her experience of many years working with many thousands of people, 'intuition is not a gift – it is a skill and it can be learned'.[10] I would go so far as to suggest (having trained in person with Dr Myss and worked with many thousands of people in movement and manual practice, as students, participants, and delegates) that it is a skill that can be restored. We might be born with it – we might have simply forgotten. We might just be 'out of touch' with our selves.

There is little doubt in my mind that if it is possible to tune in to another being, or teach someone how to do that, the ability to detect something invisible, unquantifiable, and extremely difficult to define intellectually is a most valuable asset. It is a function of time, of atten-tion, and of awareness and it starts with taking the lid off the left-brained determination to reduce (and restrict) human, multidimensional com-plexity to mechanics. We are not machines. The end.

Even if someone bases what they teach in biomechanical metaphor, that isn't what makes it work. It is their conviction and demonstration, their practice and their own charism that gives the students confidence and brings the movement protocol to life. The explanation is based in the notion that anything in the human body can be reduced to a two-bar pin joint. It resembles one in the standard iconic drawings. In engineering terms, the different classes of lever bend the wrong metaphor. There are no levers in non-linear biologic forms.

If a teacher refers to the resting point called the elbow as a 'third class lever at the olecranon process' – which is how it can be drawn to appear– that doesn't explain how it moves. The elbow folds, in a spiral configuration, as part of a sequence of myofascial tissues in complete continuity with the rest of the body.

---

10   One of Caroline Myss's themes in her classroom, where I studied Sacred Contracts in person at the CMED Institute in Chicago.

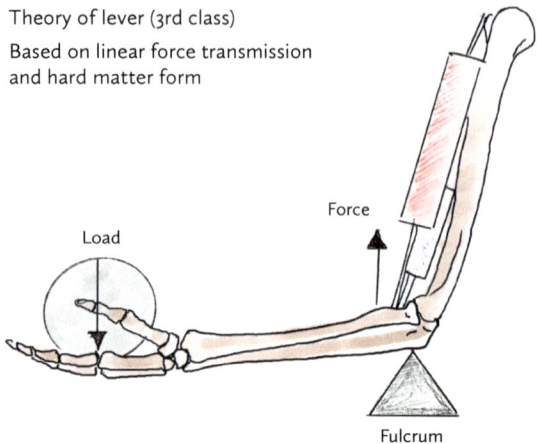

Theory of lever (3rd class)

Based on linear force transmission and hard matter form

Load

Force

Fulcrum

Figure 22

In my own practice and classes, I have noticed that each client, course participant, and student brings unique gifts and requires different styles and deliveries for the information to be incorporated in a way that works for them. Their matrix is expressive of their archetypal pattern in both soma and spirit or soul. The clearer and more congruent their body and being are, the lighter hearted and more adaptable and confident they seem to be. They move in their way; they honour their tissue improvement uniquely to their patterns.

I come across this whether teaching movement or manual therapy – or taking people through the Mapping your Archetype Profile (MAP) sequence or the MAP Somatics programme. It's too delicious and fruitful to ignore. In a way, the five Rs this book and programme are based on are five movement archetypes. They are expressed in unique ways for everyone. Rather than offering you more moves, they give you ways to honour the movements you are already trained in, so that whomever you are teaching can adapt them to *their* way. That allows each teacher to work with delicious ingredients and make the movement 'dishes' that nourish them best. Their particular flavour profiles and preferences will always be unique.

Speaking of flavour profiles, let's use this wonderful metaphor (of delicious and nourishing movement) to consider this a key metaphor that really works to help explain human motion and structure in all its variability and adaptability.

THE MAGIC OF A LIQUID CRYSTAL MATRIX

Chocolate is a liquid crystal that everyone is very familiar with, that makes perfect structural sense of how the human body forms itself and constantly renews, replenishes, and changes its shape and form. Sort of. It isn't 100% ideal (any more than a machine metaphor or a computer metaphor is) but it provides a level of insight into the way we move that levers will never reach.

Chocolate is of course organic, rather than *living,* by the time we taste it. Yet, as a metaphor, it is so often a source of sensory delight, that it's worth exploring. It resonates with the fascia as a sensory organ. It's a powerful organic metaphor, if only to shift away from machines for a moment and break the spell that they have cast over many aspects of movement practices.

ABOUT CHOCOLATE

Cacao came to Europe around the time of the Renaissance period and, like the study of the human body, it was changed irrevocably by the Industrial Revolution. Machines were made that could transform it into the food we call chocolate or couverture (at its best) and candy (at its worst). In some ways, chocolate suffered the same process of separation into its component parts as human anatomy. Colonized and eventually taken over by the commercial markets and manufacturers of processed, denatured food, this once exalted and exclusive 'food of the gods' has become a commercial product that often doesn't bear much resemblance to its original form. Despite all of this, however, the mythology and mystery of the so-called 'minor goddess' known as Ixcacao retains a magic that still holds an appeal for people. There is a resonance around the myth that somehow hasn't been lost to the ravages of time.

Ixcacao (pronounced *Ish-kak-cow*) was a goddess, her mantra was connectivity and kindness to humans. The tree, known as *Theobroma cacao*, grew typically in tropical zones either side of the equator, a creature of the 'in between' of the rain forest. The tall canopy trees, such as avocado and mango, towered over *T. cacao*, yet her beautiful fruits (when they fell to the forest floor and fermented around the beans) fed the mycelium and served that connective tissue matrix that honoured the symbiotic ecosystem of the jungle.

T. cacao grows its flowers from the trunk. They are cross-pollinated by tiny midges that thrive in such places as orchid cups and other flora and fauna in their native forests where rainwater sits at the right temperature for them to live and do their work. The flowers become the fruit of the pods, which is very delicious and wraps the 30–40 cacao beans that nestle inside its white lychee-like juicy pulp. When the pods split, the fruit ferments and transforms the beans into the first stage of the delicacy they are capable of becoming. In natural cultivation, the beans are then separated from the dried pulp, roasted, and ground. That unique combination of fermented, roasted cacao (which is cocoa powder and cocoa butter in its original form) is then mixed and whisked with water and spices and forms what has become known as 'ceremonial cacao'. That is a relatively recent term to distinguish it from the chocolate we call couverture and all kinds of variations on the theme.

The so-called ceremonial cacao contains over 200 flavour profiles and is rich in wonderful properties that have mythical stories around them. Something very delicious can happen in a gentle, ritual setting, sipping the mixture of this drink, spiced and sweetened, mimicking some of the many ways it was concocted and blended in Mayan and Aztec times. It mysteriously evokes connection and warmth in a group setting and participants somehow relax as it animates the very kindred spirit Ixcacao is known for.

During the Industrial Revolution, chocolate (which the Spanish conquistadors brought to Europe to the Baroque courts) was recognized as an elixir, highly sought-after (as were tea, coffee, and sugar) as luxurious commodities that the wealthy merchant classes, royalty, and gentry could enjoy. The beans were cultivated and grown in a less natural and more forced way on the developing plantations across the world; brought to the West via the trading routes. The European manufacturers then, eventually, developed machines that could roast and conch the beans – which they could then separate into component parts. (Divide and conquer still the abiding theme.)

The complex flavour profiles were conquered by the addition of sugar and milk powder, which further changed the original cacao into what we call couverture. That is, dark chocolate, milk chocolate, and white chocolate (which strictly speaking has no cocoa mass in it). This gave rise to a demand, among the new class of culinary experts and chocolatiers in Europe, for reliable flavour profiles. These could be achieved using different beans from different coasts and, ultimately, separating the butter and the bean to re-blend different sources of cocoa mass and cocoa butter and produce reliable flavours for the rapidly expanding chocolate market. The commercialization didn't stop there – as the discovery of the benefits of cacao butter made it valuable in its own right in cosmetics. The exquisite butter only melts at human body temperature – which makes it perfect for that market. The fat used to replace it by certain famous chocolate manufacturers was augmented (if not replaced) by vegetable fats. Indeed, there was an attempt in the twentieth century to force those factories to call it 'vegichoc' and distinguish it from real cacao and cocoa butter. That attempt failed – however, the mixture of other ingredients made 'chocolate' accessible to all. It enabled everyone to enjoy something called chocolate (even if it had scant resemblance to anything a cacao bean would recognize) and took it out to the world at affordable prices.

Cacao as a soul-food, considered by many to have a medicinal level of restorative benefits to the body, is a very different creature to couverture – what most of us know as chocolate. Like the history of anatomy, the connective tissue was removed, the body of the bean was broken down into its component parts, and the commercialized results (of chocolate and couverture) were different to the revered magical medicine of cacao.

What has *any of this* to do with the human body?

Well, from a structural point of view, it provides a metaphor way more useful and realistic in terms of structure and naturally emerging properties than a machine. The reasons for that are its organic behaviour as a liquid crystal matrix, its particular archetypal properties, its fluid dynamics, and the fact that, like fascia, it can change shape. Although it isn't living (any more than a machine is), chocolate (treated appropriately and in its original form) can also bind water. It forms an emulsion similar in some ways to our ground substance – the colloids and emulsions that make up our inner fluids.[11]

In its original legendary ritual form, cacao (appropriately roasted) can indeed bind water at the right temperature and form a heavenly drink. It forms an elixir that has survived the ravages of time for centuries, crossed cultures around the world, and even replaced money as a currency, it was considered so valuable! How mysterious is that?

The main aspect that recommends its metaphorical qualification is the way it behaves structurally in terms of emergent properties and different textures. Like fascia in the human body, chocolate is capable of presenting in a variety of forms. It can be brittle or soft, fluid or por-ridge-like in consistency. It can also change shape and incorporates the apparently magical ability to stand up by itself or blend into the shape of its container! Somehow chocolate defies being reduced to its component parts and defined or categorized as one thing. For sure there is nothing mechanical about it!

Essentially, we can appreciate the mysterious resonance of its liquid crystal behaviour, by understanding the five Ts that explain the features a chocolatier has to include in working with this wonderful organic material. Like the master chocolatier, we dance with emergent properties all the time!

Those key features are as follows: type, temporality, tempo, tempera-ture, and temper. These aspects are deeply interdependent, and all have to be taken into consideration when working with it. Chocolate, in order to take shape, has to be 'tempered'. It has to be heated and cooled in a very particular way (at a very particular temperature range for its type) to then harden into the shape of a mould. I will take the poetic license here, when likening it to the liquid crystal matrix of the human body, to use the term 'temperament' when comparing the two.

Type: There are many different types of chocolate, in a variety of colours, flavours, and mixtures. As described above, this depends on the origin, the proportions and ratios of cocoa mass to cocoa butter,

---

11   'Bodily fluids, more appropriately compared to thick paint (e.g., emulsions or colloids), are all liquid crystal matrices, including lymph, blood, mucus, cerebrospinal fluid, and synovial fluid. All reflect the variety in their viscosities along this spectrum. Notably, the ground substance of these liquid crystalline matrices is bound water.' From Sharkey, J. (2024) *Understanding Fascia, Tensegrity, and Myofascial Trigger Points: A Roadmap for Fascia-Focused Therapists.* Human Kinetics.

and the additional blends to make it palatable (as confectionery). Other additions such as sugar and milk change the appearances (which changes the behaviours!). Within the actual range of beans, however, cocoa bean blends from different countries, climates, and cultivations have distinct flavours. Each flavour will have its own optimum variables of the other four Ts. It is as carefully cultivated as any grapes for wine, or coffee beans to make a favourite espresso blend, or tea leaves to transform into tea or tisane. Each one represents a kind of alchemy, whereby the original plant is transformed into a golden elixir, with the right treatment.

Temporality: To change into the appropriate elixir or take the required shape, chocolate relies heavily on timing; both of the process and the synchronicities involved in its transformation. There are multiple heating and cooling procedures, and they all rely on dosage, degree, and the *length of time* (periodicity) at each temperature. This also depends on the specific point in the procedure and purpose for which the chocolate (and its type) is being created. Wrapping chocolate around something (such as a nut, or a piece of candied fruit, for example) is a very different timing and process to making a centre out of chocolate or moulding a chocolate 'case' into which a centre will be dosed.

Tempo: Tempo refers to the rhythm and motion and *rate of change* in working with the different processing stages. It is also about the *intervals* of change throughout the process. To turn the cocoa beans into chocolate, they have to go through certain processing (roasting, grinding, 'melanging', conching, etc.) to release the mass from the liquor; at least in what is called 'processed chocolate'. Indeed, even in the most organic way of working with 'ceremonial cacao', whisking it in water to make the elixir drink requires appropriate rhythmical movement!

The conching and melanging processes are mostly part of the industrialized use of chocolate, as it requires the releasing of certain 'unwanted volatiles' that directly affect the sought after 'flavour profile'. It also affects the size of the particles which affects, in turn, the texture of the finished couverture in fashionable culinary production of chocolate, in all its various guises. The organic, ceremonial drink is less demanding and more tolerant of the mood of the day. Cacao naturally contains complex flavour profiles (much like humans!) and these are adjusted in the recipes and blends of compatible spices and flavourings such as vanilla or chilli.

When chocolate is being made into solid confections, it is melted and treated in the various possible ways. Throughout the process, it has to be stirred continuously (it must be moved) or it just solidifies if it is in an environment cooler than its melting point. (In a working temperature higher than its melting point, it will just soften into a soggy mass of undifferentiated gloop!) The tempo of suitable motion is essential – as is an appropriate rhythm if the chocolate (at each stage) is to behave in a manageable way. At every process (and each form or morphology) it has its own viscosity, which is crucial to the success of the shape to be created. Stillness is used as a means to cool chocolate, so that it sets and becomes brittle in advance of being remelted. The time it takes to harden is the window of manipulation to achieve the desired outcome. It could be said that there is a rhythm to each stage and, if it is respected, then it contributes to the excellence of the results intended by the artisan chocolatier. It is a rhythmical, time-dependent process.

Temperature: Every type of chocolate and its component elements has to be treated at the right or optimum temperature for its type and for the stage of the process it undergoes, whether that is the cocoa butter, or the ceremonial cacao drink or some homemade Christmas treats or the manufacture of a chocolate rabbit for Easter. Each element has an optimal melting point, which is crucial to any preparation. If the right temperature is not achieved at each stage, the result will be affected.

Temper(ament): The word 'temper' refers to the heating and cooling process that is used to make metal harden and become strong. Chocolate is similar in that it also has to be tempered to form the appropriate type of architecture and textures at the different stages. This is technically referred to as the 'pre-crystalizing phase'. In terms of chocolate, it means it is heated, cooled, and re-heated. Please note it is subjected to very specific temperature variations over specific periods or intervals for each type of chocolate. This is crucial to understand because that balance facilitates the seeding and promotion of its crystalline properties (over time). That means it can adapt to (and adopt) and sustain different morphologies (shapes) when it sets.

Tempering chocolate produces what's called an 'homogenous mixture of stable and unstable crystals' with the object of the stable crystals 'overwhelming' the unstable crystals in order to eventually set into a particular crystalline matrix. (This is why the timing skills are so crucial.) The reason that unstable crystals must also be present is so that the chocolate will remain workable for whatever purpose it is being worked for. To maintain the equilibrium at each stage, the stirring (moving it) and the temperature and tempo (specific to type) maintain the workability of the chocolate. (It is temperamental material!) Melted chocolate readily becomes tempered chocolate, when a certain amount of tempered chocolate is added to it. One 'seed crystals' the other. It is a beautiful natural process that doesn't require a nervous system!

I am not saying humans are made of chocolate. I am saying that chocolate, with all its rich variable ability and alchemical mystery, gives us a way of seeing the body's liquid crystal matrix in a new metaphorical light. (At least it is a reprieve from explaining levers!) It is a light worth shining, because it actually makes more sense than a mechanical metaphor is ever going to. At least it is organic and inexplicably magical and somewhat mysterious and very variable. (Welcome to the world of humans being! Remember it is still a metaphor, although it represents human beingness somewhat more symbolically than a machine – we still are not made of cocoa beans!)

All that being said, chocolate is a wonderfully contrary and mysterious, multifaceted, complex, and variable substance. The balance of all these elements gives rise to unique structures and confections. That makes much more sense to me of adaptability and variability and diversity in human form and motion, integrated with the biomotional intelligence and nature of the being, than a machine! It remains, nevertheless, a metaphor – no more or less so than a machine or an anatomy train.

The Rs it gives us include 'regulation', 'resonance', 'relationships', 'recognition' and 'recreation', to mention a few that raise our understanding of the physical nature of our ingenious matrix. If it helps, even in a small way, to unify beings with their bodies, so they can enjoy *being them*, it's worth considering! (Especially when we discover delicious movement!)

In the next part of the book, we will examine the element of magic that myofascia also resonates with. Rather than the more esoteric Rs that could be included, the focus will be on the five physical ones that *animate* our liquid crystal matrix and revitalize it. They are designed to restore (at progressively subtle levels) the innate properties of our biomotional intelligence – the one our myofascial matrix relies upon to signal to us from the inside, if only we will tune in, listen, and recognize its sensory subtleties. Whatever the movement modality you are trained in, awareness of these fundamental five Rs will deepen and enhance the difference it already makes. The history each practitioner has accumulated can be honoured more with the mystery and magic added back into the movement practice! (Even if you approached your training from a mechanical point of view – you can take it to new levels if you recognize the non-mechanistic nature of the form you are trained to help move better!)

Please note, in Chapter 7 of *Yoga Fascia and Movement* there is more detail on this theme. It includes the vast subject of bound water – looking at research from Gerald Pollack and Mae Wan Ho, to mention only two of the scientists who have devoted their lives to understanding the liquid crystal nature of bound water. It is far more than a form. Their work includes the essential understanding of the electromagnetic field of living water – at the interfaces of the tissues and cells. It is beyond the scope of this book and will come into the series of books this one is part of. At this point, it is enough to shift from the old metaphor of machines to the new one of liquid crystal matrices. I'm not surprised – I love that science is catching up with the wisdom of the ancients – if nothing else, it restores magic and mystery to its rightful place in the being of humanity.

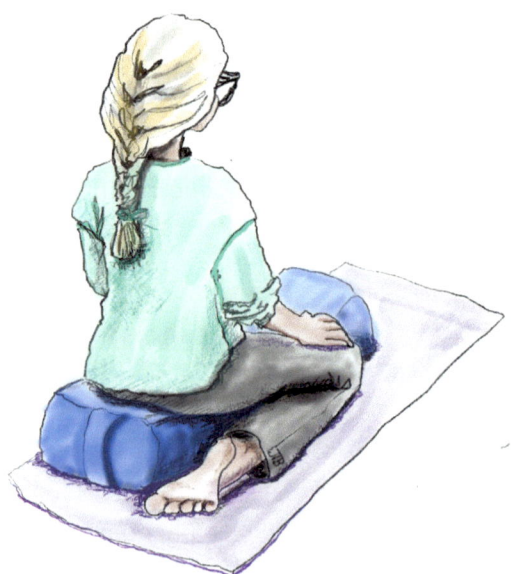

Figure 23 Angela Farmer quoted 'Better one's own dharma followed imperfectly than another's dharma perfectly done. Better to die than to follow another's dharma.'[12]

12   In class on retreat in Greece with Angela Farmer, quoting from the Bhagavad Gita according to Krishna, 'it is better to do one's own dharma imperfectly than another's perfectly'. (Dharma can be translated as 'purpose'.)

BREATH BY JOANNA CRUICKSHANKS

I move in the shapes of people. bones, tissue
pulsate imperceptibly beneath
fixed minds of identity.
sages crowned me spirit of all that is long before modern anatomy
minimized me to an inflow and outflow system – a chemical
concoction to fuel the pump mechanism of bodily machines.
everything in nature threaded through the needle-eye-mind of a culture
obsessed by breaking it all down. one eye closed. the other squinting.
I am more than a tidy morsel of understanding, more
than a respiratory function. my place is in metabolizing
mystery out there to remember what is within.
the silence knows.
pneuma. In-spirit-us.
extractive minds miss movements of life's
meandering
marvellously
there is no line here
no simple in and out
we are all more than our mechanics
I breathe you, not you me
unseen an-in-ma
I am not an in-and-out thing
I circle, encircle, dissolve,
enliven, inspire, and expire...
the last one
woven with all past last ones
will find its way into freshly
born flesh.
buds and sacs expand bodaciously to my arrival.
to life meeting life
to each breath whirling and swirling its invisible thread down
through the lungs, into each cell and back out to meet green
this is life's dance
an endless crochet of breath threads passing from
and through – back to the nothingness
warp weft. body breath.
I contain in me

all the stories of last ones
becoming the first ones.
I whisper life's great mystery into each cell.
it's all one big breath
moving us through.
Shapeshifting, space weaving, infinite ebb and flow.

Part 3

THE MAGIC

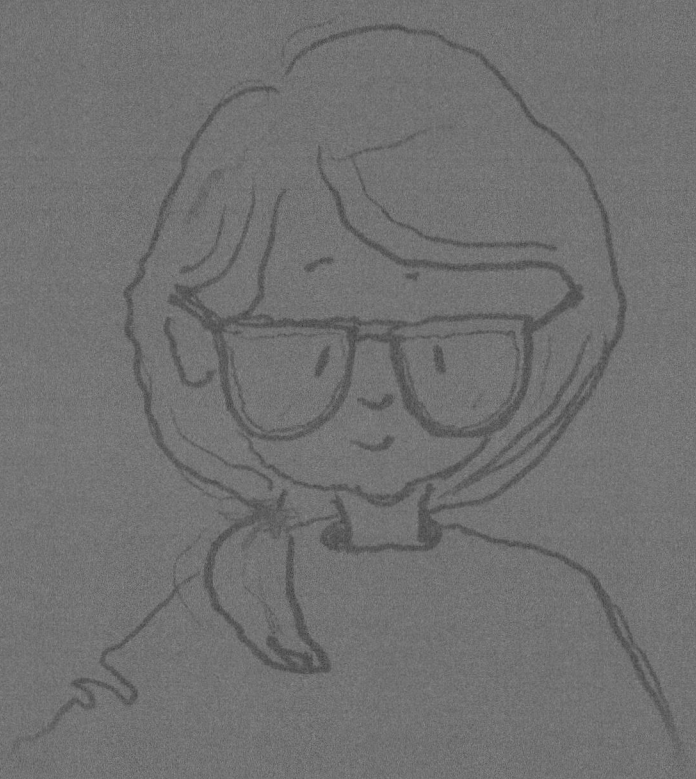

Human body architecture is a miraculous and magical organization that has been misunderstood and misrepresented for centuries. It is that simple and that complex!

Understanding fascia (and the myofascial magic it provides access to) is crucial to recognizing that the body-wide nature of the living structure is far more intelligent, detailed and significant than almost anyone understood in previous ages. Many modalities dismiss it as a fad. However, the science and the spirit of the scientific questions (not to mention all the experiences and research from practitioners and authors and protagonists in the field) urge everyone to wake up. Thomas Hanna refers brilliantly in his work to something called 'somatic amnesia'. The magical thing about understanding fascia is that it fundamentally awakens each being to the home it resides in. I might use somewhat different explanations than others (see the author contributions in this book) and somewhat different methods to animate them (see the practices in this book), however, many of us are coming from the same heart-centred place. It is something about awakening to the inner sense of sensory innerness. Whatever it's called, the process of unifying is magical!

That inner sense, and the 'internal net highways' of the fascia it travels on, serves us 24/7. Working to animate, recognize, and remember it (appreciate and revere it), helps us to know ourelves better and access our well-being as a daily resource. If someone takes supplements, it isn't for an instant fix. It is to ongoingly support an ingredient that assists the body to express itself with resilience and appropriate resonance over time. These Rs (resonance, resilience, resource, and so on) are the results of the physical five Rs of myofascial magic (see Part 5). They support the treasure inside each one of us, that can be called upon so we can respond appropriately at the time.

When listening to the radio and tuning in to a favourite kind of music, there is no orchestra inside the radio box. It is an antenna with appropriate aerial and inner workings and amplification to resound with the acoustics or audio waves that it has been tuned into. The same goes for the music in a smartphone, or any app for that matter. There is no artist, singer, mathematician or blank page in the phone or tablet. There is huge possibility and the right sounds and haptics settings, with suitable memory and the appropriate display on the liquid crystal interface on the screen, to *interface* with any one of the apps and *become* the musician, artist, or author as a result. Depending on how we interact with them, the rest is up to the user! Think of fascia as *something like* the apps, the interface, and the user all integrated. It forms the structure, filters the food, transmits the forces, contains the energy, guards the shapes, communicates the messages and interfaces the light, sound, and touch that makes it into something each one creates. If there is something magical about what can be achieved with a smart phone or tablet, then know that such resources exist within the human body being, if only it knew! No mechanics required.

HUMAN MAGICAL INGREDIENTS

Humans being have three particularly magical ingredients within their living, architectural matrix. They are *structure, somasense,* and *spirit*. I call them magical because they remain mysterious (they reveal themselves at the right time, in the right space) and they don't behave mechanically or to order (they respond accordingly) and, most importantly, they are unique to each one of us. How very inconvenient, unpredictable and wonderfully human!

Structure: the optimal organization, or design, our species generally expresses (given that unique variations are the norm) contains a magical feature that is free. It is our innate elastic recoil or 'free energy storage capacity' to give it a technical name. Let's call it 'spring'. It is what elite athletes foster to perform at peak structural efficiency. It is what people (most people) can spend just minutes a day resourcing. We inadvertently deprive this ability (we effectively stratify and stupefy it) when we sit for hours, lean forward for hours, or slowly impose a repetitive strain injury in the body posture or structure (over time) without necessarily realizing or consciously relieving it. Over time it has an impact on the structure. In very small amounts of time, it can often eventually be changed. Transformation is a thing a human body can often do in good time.

Somasense is not separate from structure. Fascia forms the structure and contains the fluid matrix (or liquid crystal matrix) that it is. It is also the sensory organ we are describing. In this context, somasense is our 'fascia feedback sensory awareness system' which is, in and of itself, a unique and personal resonance field. They are not separate (nothing is).

Somatic sensory awareness, or somasense, is closely related to something more formally described as proprioception. It is often referred to as the 'sixth sense', however, I believe it to be our primary sense as it is how each and every embryo feels its way into form. Proprioception is considered to comprise interoception (internal) and exteroception (external). While we come into our own self-awareness (which is what proprioception really invites) we can follow the 'multiply up and unite' trend, rather than 'divide and conquer' by breaking proprioception down into more details. The fascia matrix is constantly balancing internal and external forces around and through us and for us. It does that anyway – possibly way beyond anything the thinking mind can get its reasoning around. It isn't reasonable. It is a little mysterious and a lot magical. (That's not a licence to be unscientific, it is simply pointing out that the intellectual aspect of this is not the only one. It is about beings in bodies that have instinctive, moving responses, and intuitive ones, too. Every one arrives as a whole).

Spirit is the third magical ingredient, in the spirit of the occasion, the place, the time, the space, the being and the Grace. The unaccountable, unquantifiable, qualia we each experience. If we wanted to assign a 'who' to those aspects of us, this might be called (softly) the basic self, the conscious self, and the high self. They could be considered three key 'managing agents' within each of us that influence how we do things in the physical world around us (the basic self), how we interface physical and metaphysical (the conscious self) and how we animate both and express them for the highest good (the high self) as congruently as possible. It's a bigger conversation (beyond the scope of this book), however, it makes sense of a particular asset of the fascial matrix that must not be lost to the way we study the body. It is all one within every body. That oneness is animated by the spirit. There's no need to break that down into its component parts, either. Suffice to say here that it's what makes you do you the way you do it, me do me the way I do and them do them the way they do. It's the movement of spiritual inner awareness that guides and drives every body.

This part of the book will look at all three of these magical ingredients, with emphasis on the structure. Together they form a foundation of biomotional intelligence. It is available to everyone. The practice (in Part 5) raises the resonance naturally, of the structure, the somasense, and the spirit, without thinking about it. It simply requires doing. Like everything that works, there is an aspect of the techniques that remains mysterious! The results are magical. That, too, is part of being human.

Who would imagine that a tiny amount of appropriate micro-movements could transform a severe surgical insult into a relative non-issue in 12 weeks, with less than 12 minutes a day of refined movement practices from the five Rs described in this book? This author's experience, after major surgery, was that despite the opportunity for chording, and tethering from scar tissue, it is possible to go from zero range of motion to completely restored in this time period.

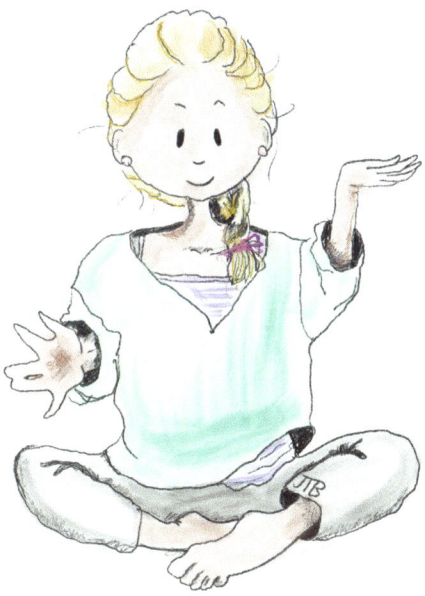

Figure 24

STRUCTURE

It is not only in the field of anatomy, physiology, posture, and structure that the influence of a mechanical metaphor can be considered to have underserved the general understanding of the body and how it moves! (Not to mention how it 'feels' its way into form.) Neuroscientist David Perlmutter, for example, made the following statement in a podcast in 2023 with Ranjan Chattergee:

We still labour through this dichotomy between the health of the brain and the health of the body as if there is some division...and this gets back to Descartes and the whole notion of systems...and looking at the body as a machine; the brain being the computer, the heart is the pump, the lungs are the bellows and there should be no interaction. You know the reality of it all is that the body functions as an integrated whole.

(David Perlmutter, neuroscientist)[1]

Perhaps one of the key contributors to this deep issue lies in the most basic understanding of how the embryo forms. It will require another book (later in this series), however, the foundation of recognition that every human being feels its way into form, via the intrinsic architecture of the fascia matrix, *as a whole*, changes the basis of how movement is understood as an expression of that whole form. All the time. What we move *and what we do not move*, are expressions of the whole, the whole time. Recognizing that changes everything we thought we knew!

FREE ENERGY STORAGE CAPACITY

Have you ever seen someone spring lightly up onto a step or three, from standing? (You've most likely seen a cat bound easily upward from a standing start!) Have you seen a climber leap or swing across a climbing wall, with no more than their toes and fingertips holding onto the rock protrusions, springing their whole-body weight up or across the wall-face? How do they do that? Have you seen someone holding their body inside a giant hoop while it rolls around the floor, or holding a vertical stick planted in the ground, with their hands, while their torso and legs are held out parallel to the ground? Perhaps you have seen examples of marvellous partner performances, where both bodies move as one continuum, balancing and extending out from the smallest area of contact? Maybe you have watched the Olympics and seen an elite athlete

1   Chattergee, R. (Host) (2023, June 7) The Key Driver of Chronic Disease That Nobody's Talking About with David Perlmutter (No. 368) [Audio podcast episode] In *Feel Better, Live More*. Acast. https://podcasts.apple.com/gb/podcast/feel-better-live-more-with-dr-rangan-chatterjee/id1333552422?i=1000615884929

running in slow motion, seemingly airborne for longer than they touch the track? Or a basketball player appear to hang suspended in the air for a nanosecond and drop the ball into the net, ten feet or more above the ground?

Do you wonder how any of these examples are even possible when we are supposedly made of stacked bones, balancing one on top of the other, with a spinal 'column' up the middle, supporting our heads from underneath? Do we have to be super fit 'pillars of strength' to achieve such feats? How on earth does a body of 50–100 kg spring across a climbing wall, holding on (with that amount of weight) by the tiny muscles of the fingertips and toes? The most basic biomechanical laws do not account for it.

Is there another ingredient that we don't always account for? Could it be something available to the human body design that we could all tap into – at least in small doses – deep within our structure? Not just the fit, the strong or the elite athletes, but all of us?

The answers to these and many of the riddles behind apparently extraordinary human actions (especially the ones that seem to defy gravity), lie in something deeply misunderstood about the way we (and other animals) form. It is a force available to every single one of us, to a greater or lesser extent because of the way we each self-organized as embryos.

Is it possible that, even if we have no desire to roll around inside a hoop or join the circus as a trapeze artist, we could simply walk with a lighter step and 'bounce back' more easily if and when we stumble?

We are formed under very particular patterns that give us our volume. Those patterns mean we all have this magical ingredient called 'spring'. How we tap into it, resource it, and treasure it is the question this book is based on.

This is a side-teach that will be detailed far more fully in the next book in the series, *Fasciategrity in Motion*. Here we can simply outline the foundation of this essential piece about living structure and the magic ingredient that fasciategrity provides. It explains that the body is 'one' (and it is explained *by* that). The human design contains its own dynamic structure and that is the basis of its biomotional intelligence and integrity, physically, emotionally, and spiritually, given that the anima/animus that expresses each person, uniquely to them, is in motion. No one survives *being themselves* without this, yet it was hidden behind the 'hard matter' physics applied through the wrong metaphor!

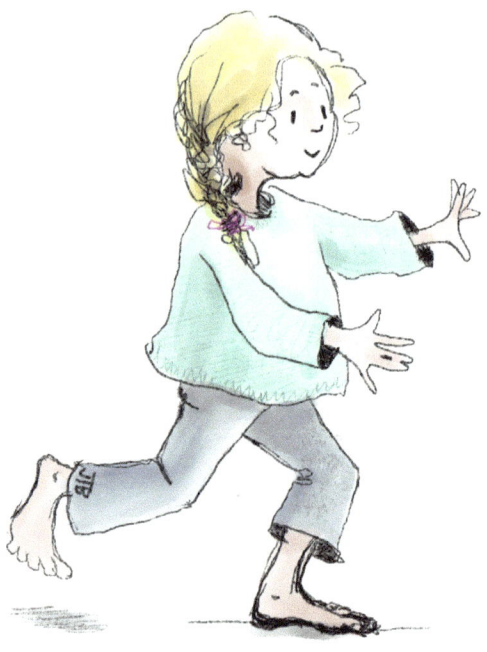

Figure 25

Fasciategrity: our structural dynamics ('spring')

We all formed 'under tension'. That means something like how an umbrella stays up when you click it open. We've already uncovered how we are made of soft matter – and, of course, the umbrella is made of hard matter – but this metaphor is useful to demonstrate something very important. The umbrella's components are not living in constant flux, nor can they move by themselves as humans can. However, they do hold their shape, by the organization of two forces in a particular reciprocal pattern. That particular pattern is what is being explored here, in the umbrella, before distinguishing it in the human body design.

The two forces holding the umbrella open are tension (think of the fabric) and compression (think of the spokes) when they work together. The organization of the structure is a very specific design that balances these two forces in a very particular way. It is called a 'tension compression architecture'. The umbrella has a pole up the middle, with a holding button to maintain that particular tension–compression structural pattern in place. (Note, it is not living, moving or responding; it is a static example of this architectural pattern). The umbrella is, of course, open underneath and we have to hold the pole the correct way up for it to do its job (and pray the wind doesn't turn it inside-out) while it protects us from the rain. The umbrella can then be closed (by releasing the tension–compression holding structure) and folded away until it is needed again. Everything in that structure relies on the way it is joined together. It is complex, but it works to change function by changing shape and restoring it, based on its particular design and structural organization.

Another example of a tension–compression structure is the marquee you enter when you go to the circus. While you sit watching the wonderful trapeze artists swinging through the air or the acrobats performing the feats we described earlier, you rely on the tension–compression architecture of the tent to stay open in a volume around you. Much like the umbrella, it has tensional canvas or fabric and compressional poles to organize it. The marquee also has adjustable guy wires attaching it to the ground outside and at least one central mast holding it up in the middle. The marquee (somewhat like a spider's web) must be anchored to the outside world, despite needing its inner structure of tent poles, to maintain the integrity of the internal space, or volume.

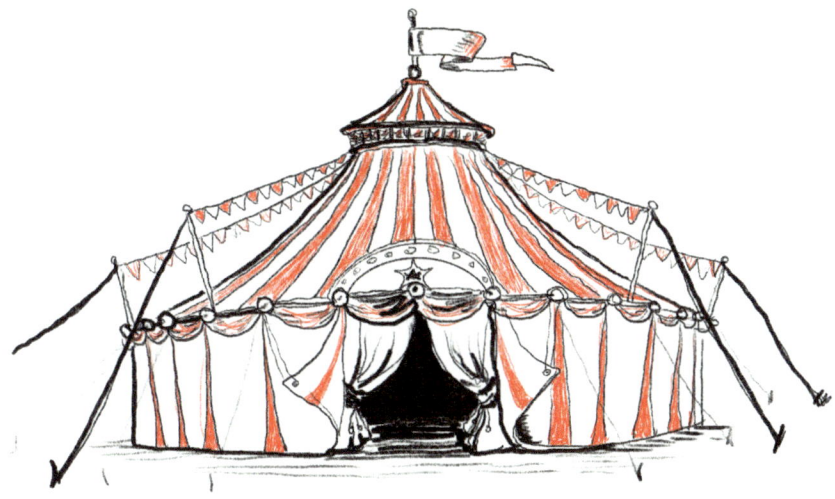

Figure 26

A spider weaves its poles and wires out of one material, but the shape and organization has tension–compression elements at the heart of its structural integrity. In both cases, an outside frame is required. What the web example helps us understand is how both tension and compression forces can be provided by pattern and organization, out of one material. (The spokes and cross-threads play both roles, however, the majority of the compression is provided by the frame.) The web has an outside anchor from the bushes, or corners of the room to which it attaches, and the spider tensions the web as a surrounding resonance field to live in. It knows which threads are not sticky – unlike the unfortunate fly that gets caught for its breakfast. The spider also knows (through the vibration of the web) whether a mate waits patiently for attention (knowing they don't know which threads are sticky) or a fly awaits it as breakfast, stranded by the threads and reacting violently to the trap. Webbing is smart material! It resonates!

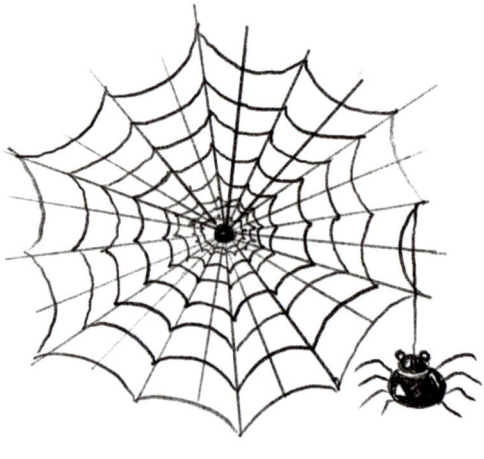

Figure 27

Another example used in literature to explain tension–compression architecture is that of a mast on a boat, with a sail attached to it that is tensioned by the stays (ropes at the back of the boom anchored to the boat) and the sheets (ropes) attached to the sail and the boat. In a manner of speaking, this is more like a different version of the umbrella principle. Like the marquee, the mast must be attached to something for basic stability (the deck of the boat) and like the umbrella, the sail has to be able to fill with wind (changeably) and be held down at the same time. It is indeed another type of tension–compression architecture and relies on similar structural principles.

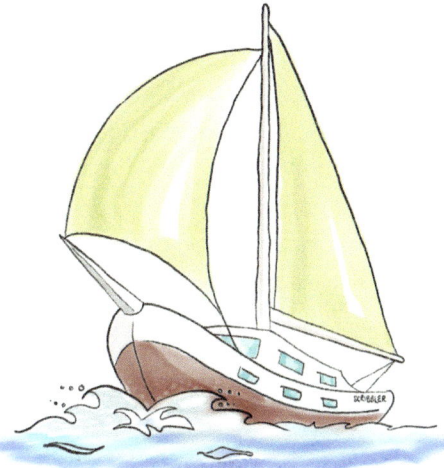

Figure 28

A wheel can take us to the next level of complexity. A wagon wheel is purely a compression structure. Although it is round and designed as a wheel, it doesn't rely on any tension to speak of to hold its structure. A bicycle wheel, however, incorporates tension and compression within its design. In fact, with a minimum of 12 spokes (providing tension) and a rim and hub (providing compression), it qualifies as a particular type of tension–compression architecture. It is a tensegrity structure because it needs no outside frame. Unlike the marquee, the boat, or the spider's web, the bicycle wheel does not lose its integrity or structure when it isn't fixed to the bike or anything else around it.

You and I are different from all the above – we live at the next level of complexity because we are not just 'round' like the circular wheel. We are whole rounded volumes, taking 'spherical' to the next level of tubular and mobile. Wherever we are on the scale of ability and agility, we have our entire 'frame, mast, poles, webs, guy wires, hubs, and rims' on the inside. We move them around with us because, unlike the tent, the web, the boat, the umbrella, or the bicycle wheel, we are closed and fully enclosed structures, wherever we are. Those internal 'poles and guy wires' are somewhat like our bones and tendons, holding us as volumes, wrapped in the fabric of our skin or tissue sheaths and enclosed and held open by our diaphragms and dynaments.[2] We don't deflate. We remain, like the umbrella, 'up and open' in the sense that we stay fully up and we stay round, even if we are lying down. We adapt. Unlike the umbrella, we don't have a hemispherical design – we are rounded. We are contained, in the round, surrounding our own frames.

We are not even circular (like the wheel), but variously tubular structures on every scale. Our vessels, our limbs, our torso, and neck are all tubes of varying thicknesses. Even our guts, ligaments, and hearts rely on tubular forms, spiralling into form.

We can fold and unfold, but we don't collapse. We stay rounded. We remain as volumes in every position. We don't completely close up and fold away, like the umbrella or the marquee. We can soften and stiffen, but we don't 'empty the air or the contents out' and fold down like a flat-packed tent, squished into a bag after a camping trip. We keep the appropriate spaces, too, such as those that guard the nerves from the spinal cord, or the openings at the nostrils and ears (the foramen), whatever position we are in. Our limbs, torso, and head are rounded, tubular shapes as are all the tubes and tissues and vessels within us. They can fold down to an extent (like our bladder folds when it's empty and fills and expands until we empty it again) but that's a shape change with a limit.

In order to remain able to shape change and integrate within all the other aspects of our moving body, everything in us must be formed under tension, in complete continuity with everything else in the body. The technical name for our living structure is a 'pre-tensioned' or a 'pre-stiffened' architecture. You could say it means that we (in relation to a metaphorical umbrella) stay opened out – if not exactly 'up' – all the time! The respiratory diaphragm is the best example. It isn't separate from the heart and lungs above it, or the abdominal organs below it, but it remains like the open umbrella, moving between the upper and lower aspects of the tubular torso, shape changing in a suitable rhythm without releasing that tension *with every breath*.

2   See Avison, *Yoga, Fascia, Anatomy and Movement*, Chapter 3: 'Jaap van der Wal coined the term "dynament" as an inclusive name that better represents the muscle–tendon–bone–ligament–synovial joint relationship from a functional, *architectural* point of view, given the tissue continuity he established at every joint in the body.' He suggests that to use or label *a "synovial joint"* [as such] *is a contradiction in terms. It is not a joint. It is a dis-joint. Here connective tissue (cartilage) enables space and therefore motion*' (Jaap van der Wal in a private communication).

Think about that for a moment. Your diaphragm has been something like an open umbrella every day of your life since you formed it embry-onically. In the earliest stage of your heart-centred spine-design, it was forming across the torso while your heartbeat syncopated the whole orchestrated, body-forming symphony![3] The diaphragm is in synch with everything around it, because it isn't separate, in structure or fabric. The heart rests on it. The diaphragm is only different in texture, density, and *type* of tension–compression organization and shape. This is somewhat like a variation on the idea (metaphorically) of the open umbrella inside us: always 'up' but able to fill and flow the air by changing shape as we breathe in and breathe out, in concert with everything else. These are relatively small ranges of motion within our living anatomy.

Our lungs don't fully fill or fully empty. They grow (inhale) and let go (exhale) either side of their 'resting tension' at around 50% full.

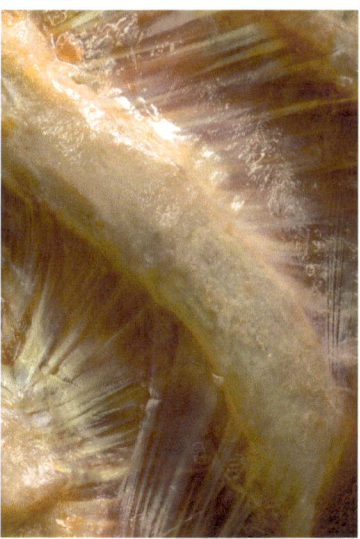

Figure 29 Image of rib fascia.
With permission from John Sharkey.

---

3   See Avison, *Yoga, Fascia, Anatomy and Movement*, Chapter 4: The Remarkable Human Blueprint.

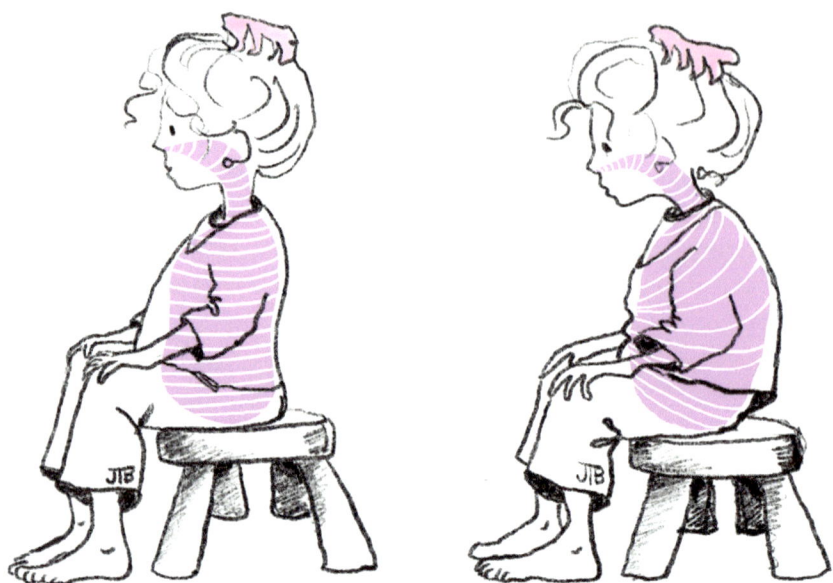

Figure 30

Everything in the body structure is 'spring loaded' by its nature, contained within the tubular torso, where it first formed in the embryo
under tension. Everything is either under more or less tension, or more
or less compression, in co-creative balance. It's a 'both/and' story of the
whole body, from our beginning to our last breath. Everything moves
everything else moving *all the time*. Our ability to modify and *only do*
something specific and appear to *only use* the parts we need, is a triumph
of organization, coordination, and fasciategrity! It is structural brilliance
displayed persistently with every breath we take and move we make. It is
the ability to pick up a glass and drink from it without dropping it, while
using the 'other limbs' to be still and pouring *just what we need* to swallow
while returning it to the table and talking to a friend, without wearing
the drink! It is sitting in a chair interacting with a book or a tablet while
appearing not to involve the rest of the body. That is a *natural* performance. The stillness in the 'rest of the body' is an artform. Like much
to do with understanding fascia, it hides in the obvious as our innate
genius. Stillness is an asset. Poise might be the highest performance we
have. We already do that, if we can.

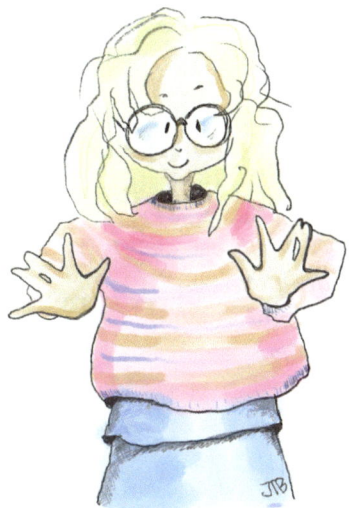

Figure 31

If you spread your hands as 'stiffly open' as you can, you will see the tendons on the backs of them resemble umbrella spokes. As an embryo, when your limbs were originally growing (after your torso had formed with the diaphragm across it), they grew from buds out of the torso. The innermost part (that was eventually going to become bone) grew considerably faster than the outermost part (that was already becoming skin). The muscles and tissues in between them (such as tendons, nerves, and blood vessels) all became tensioned, to a greater or lesser extent, partly by this growing pattern and the different rates of growth within each limb. (Each type of tissue is a type of fascia, growing at its own rate.) That means, structurally, you are organized from the inside out, to maintain your shape without external support. Ideally, there is an optimal balance between the two forces of tension and compression. It changes according to scale and motion; we 'phase change'. That balance is what those fabulous movement artists and athletes rely on. To varying extents, we all do, even if we can't balance perfectly upside down in a one-handed stand with our limbs in a star shape.

THE SAME PRINCIPLE GOVERNS ALL HUMAN MOTION

We can't all perform the way the athletes or the artists do. Sometimes our structure simply doesn't have certain capabilities; we are all unique expressions of that structural integrity. When something in the structure doesn't fully organize in synchrony and sympathy with the whole potential, we 'measure' that in our culture on a scale of 'ability to disability'. Sometimes there is too much stiffness in one of the fabrics and not enough in the other. Sometimes the nerve or blood vessels don't organize optimally. In other cases, the tissues are simply too soft to organize uprightness. Thinking of the umbrella as a structural metaphor, we know that if the fabric is too big for the spokes, or the spokes are not sturdy enough for the fabric, there is an imbalance in the overall architecture, and it won't work quite as well as it's designed to.

Humans and animals are each essentially made of one fabric, namely fascia, so it has to have all sorts of variations to provide all the expressions from hardest soft matter (bones) to softest soft matter (superficial fascia, under the skin, which is like egg white). We will go into this fascinating aspect of our structure in another book devoted to what we call fasciategrity.[4] It is the source (and the sauce) of the magic ingredient available to all of us, in motion.

Technically, that magic ingredient is known as 'stored energy capacity' or 'elasticity'. To keep it super simple and clear to us in terms of movement, it's basically 'bounce' in its simplest description. The essential value of this stored energy capacity is that it's free! It doesn't cost us energy, it provides it. That's magical when you have access to it!

FREE ENERGY

There is a lot of misunderstanding around both these terms. Stored energy capacity is constantly changing and elasticity is often considered synonymous with stretchy fabric (e.g., elastic). On the contrary, elasticity has very little to do with your tissues behaving like elastic bands. Steel has higher elasticity than rubber, which can seem confusing at first.

---

4   Sharkey, J. and Flannigan, M. (2023) 'Towards a paramedical interdisciplinary definition of fascia supporting practitioners offering fascia-focused therapies.' (Part 1). *International Journal of Anatomy and Applied Physiology* 9, 1, 218–222.

Let's unravel this enough to clarify why this magical ingredient is often missed or messed up. We have something in our tissues called elastin and it is often confused as our source of elasticity – it isn't. (It doesn't provide elasticity. Rebound or recoil is down to sufficient stiffness of the collagen.)

There's lots more on this in two of the chapters in *Yoga, Fascia, Anatomy and Movement* – The Elastic Body and The Elastic Breath.[5] It's a huge subject. We don't breathe with separate breathing muscles; it's just a nice idea. Studying this way can help to augment certain aspects of breathwork. However, when the whole system is regulated, it self-regulates. No one would sleep if it was an intellectual process. It's a natural process and, as such, it relies heavily on the elasticity and compliance of all the tissues. They are made of fascia under tension. If the tension–compression relationship is disharmonious, so is the compliance of the breath!

Steel ball bearings scattered over a floor will bounce everywhere without any batteries to drive them. So will rubber balls. Technically, the steel will bounce further and bounce back further than the rubber. That is why the guy wires of the marquee or the mast on a boat are made of steel rather than rubber. Steel has higher stiffness. Rubber is usually too soft to contain the optimum 'tensile strength' to manage the 'compression forces' of the wind on a craft. They both have elasticity – it can just be counterintuitive to realize that the stiffer steel has the highest elastic recoil capacity or 'energy storage capacity'.

Stored energy capacity is literally 'free energy'. It is what a kangaroo relies on to build momentum and reach leaps of more than 20 metres, travelling without exhausting itself with the sheer force transmission it manages over relatively huge distances (compared to a toad, who is using the same kind of energy over much smaller areas!) It is what a whirligig beetle relies on to spring from lily pad to pond surface. It is how a butterfly unfolds and bursts its beautiful body out of a tiny chrysalis or how a flycatcher flicks out its tongue to catch its breakfast. It is how the

5   Avison, *Yoga, Fascia, Anatomy and Movement*, Part 2.

prokaryotic cells James Oschman wrote about can move around without a nervous system.[6] It is how you and I can learn to do a cartwheel (if we ever wanted to!) without our heads falling off or our internal organs getting scrambled or spilled. That is how our structure is organized. It's already ingenious.

Your tissues have a huge variety of 'tensile strengths'. Fascia in the lumbar spine can show the tensile strength of steel,[7] while in other areas of the body it can act more like rubber or nylon thread or cling film, than steel guy wires. It includes exceptional range and variability to accommodate the range and variability of our movements. It's like a super intelligent smart fabric that can adapt to our use of it. Everywhere in the body, fascial structures are essentially contained to support and store that 'energy capacity'. It's metabolically free, so the body is fundamentally designed to preserve it wherever it can.

The head (particularly the cranial bones) is a bony chamber or container, within which the brain is wrapped in a bag. The rib basket contains the thorax and the abdominal wall and pelvis contain the visceral organs. Within those, our lungs are held in tissue pockets (pleura), the heart is held in a tissue pocket (pericardium), and the organs and gut tubes are all inside their own sacs, contained by another pocket (peritoneum). Everything inside us is folded in tubes, pockets, and pouches that wrap and connect the *one* piece of fabric of which we are made, folded and enfolded as embryos in order to form ourselves.

All this containment has a structural role in holding us together. It also compresses what is inside it and is tensioned by what is outside of it. That balance of forces changes all the time and allows us to manage our movements without collapsing or bursting. It does it so instinctively and intuitively that most of our predecessors missed it. They were analysing the parts by cutting up the wholeness that contained them. That wholeness relies on being whole to honour those forces and 'phase changes', as they are called.

Think of a balloon. As soon as you 'pop' the tensioned skin (which is compressing the air inside it) you lose the volume. When it isn't whole, it is no longer a balloon. When it's left whole long enough to leak air,

---

6   Oschman, J. L. (2012) 'Fascia as a Body-Wide Communication System.' In Schleip, R., Findley, T. W., Chaitow, L. and Huijing, P. A. (eds) *Fascia: The Tensional Network of the Human Body*. Edinburgh: Churchill Livingstone.

7   Juhan, D. (1987) *Job's Body*. New York, NY: Station Hill Press.

there's less and less to compress and the balloon goes flaccid and soft, untensioned by the inner 'pressing' of the air inside (that is pushing out, as the skin pushes in), optimal tension–compression is compromised. We actually experience tension–compression structures all the time and often miss this crucial aspect of our forming because it is so innate to us.

> Think of the balloon when you blow it up, then let go before tying the knot to keep the air in. The process of the air escaping moves the balloon randomly around the room if you let go of it. It doesn't have a battery, nor does it need an outside force to move it. The rapid change in tension–compression balance *releases the energy to move it.* It is driven by *stored energy capacity.*

One reason this aspect of our structure is termed 'energy storage capacity' is that it is innate to our design, and it is 'stored' in the way our tissues are formed. In other words, our pre-tensioned structure is the basis of this free energy. They all contain each other (the frame, the strings, the different structures we described before), while they all remain connected. It is remarkable to discover the exquisite organization of our own continuously connected bioorganic origami. Just as energy is released (as a popping sound) when the balloon bursts, so our energy is released if we know how to store and restore it in the first place – in our structure. It is innate to our design.

FREE TRAVEL

One way to imagine how tension and compression (or fasciategrity in our bodies) give us this free energy is to think of a catapult or a bow and arrow. When you use either of these gadgets, they have to be suitably tensioned by pulling on the compression aspect of the bow or catapult. The soft string is 'pulled into tension' by the holding of the stiff v-stick or the bow 'resisting with compression' in a particular shape (neither are completely rigid). The archer draws back the string and releases the arrow – or the stone if it's the catapult. They don't push the arrow, nor is it pulled from the bow. The arrow, or the stone, do not contain any battery or outside means of propulsion. The energy with which they travel on their trajectory is released. They are essentially travelling on free energy storage capacity, which comes from the structure of the bow or the catapult.

The bow and the catapult both require someone to hold them and use them for them to function (third force of movement). Once we are old enough to balance and run around (we take a bit longer to find our feet than most four-legged animals), we don't require anything outside of us to travel on this energy. We release it all over the place just by moving because of our innate structure. *We are the archer, the bow, and the arrow.* All three are required!

We already formed the harder parts and the softer parts of these potential structures within us. We already have the folds and the fabric and the poles and the guy wires, and we enfold all of them completely. That is what makes us 'living tensegrity architectures'. It is what gives us this incredible resource of 'fasciategrity' as free energy. It really is the magic ingredient of the myofascia, which is always and in all ways under tension when we are healthy. If not, we are in deep trouble. When that tensional integrity is broken – either because we break a bone, snap a tendon, or tear a muscle – the entire structure is compromised. We can't bounce! We lose the 'spring in our step' (if it's a leg injury) or the ability to 'spread our wings' (if it's an arm injury), literally and symbolically. One site of damage affects the whole. (Certain conditions lower the tension–compression balance and integration and it directly affects the ability to 'spring' or move naturally).

If compression forces overwhelm tension or tensional forces overwhelm compression, integrity is compromised. We embrace both and use both in what's called a 'co-creative force transmission'. The third aspect which facilitates movement requires the tensional force to move and the compressional force to offer suitable resistance. The balance changes with every move. Myofascial magic in action works because of these deep organizations in our tissues. It enhances the powerful, harmonic relationship between tension and compression within us, that is there in spite of everything. We form on the basis of these two forces in combined balance. That combined balance is the third force we rely upon. It cannot be separated – it is the result of our structure. Once we know how to harness and store it, we have the magic ingredient.

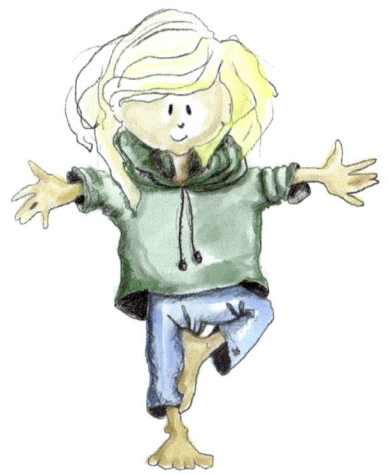

Figure 32

DOING DOES IT

One key to this is to see that, as newborn babies, we are all soft matter, and a huge percentage of our structure is fluid. We are too soft to stand up. The balance of tension and compression is still there, but its bias is too far on the 'soft' end of the spectrum; we are too malleable at this stage. We learn to organize ourselves with more and more containment as we go from baby to toddler. As we grow older and move around, we move forces through our whole bodies and our bodies respond to them accordingly. The force transmission through the fascia animates this living tissue to respond, according to our design. (That is our original species genetics.) We organize bones as we grow and gradually the soft tissues we are made of take on roles depending on where they are and how we use them. We can train ourselves into shapes that optimize our structure and the things we can do with it. If we have the ability to teach it to dance, we can dance. If we have the ability to teach it to run, we can run. We dance by dancing. We run by running. Even if we teach ourselves, we become able to do it by doing it.

That structure we form into is predicated on the ability to respond to forces, to a greater or lesser extent. It must detect the subtle and the strong, the hot from the cold, the sticky from the slippery, the dull from the bright, the rough from the smooth, moment to moment, and movement to movement. At the other end of the spectrum from the baby, we can lose our mobility and variability by becoming too dehydrated and losing that fluidity to too many of the stiffer components. As we age, we can lose that structural integrity (and very often we don't need to). We also don't need to age to lose it. Notwithstanding injury and dysfunction, we can sometimes move the needle by *not* doing and doing differently.

We can gradually sacrifice the spring for a slump. Both the spring and the slump train the tissue accordingly, so it responds by springing less and slumping more. Both are habitual patterns. We can give up our ability to bounce for more sedentary pursuits and eventually we will become that sedentary person.

Nevertheless, we are still designed with an innate structural spring loading; it is our free energy storage capacity. However, if a kangaroo spends its life in a cage, there is a fair likelihood that it won't keep up with its wild siblings on being released. If it doesn't use its legs, it will have to relearn to cover distance by having the distance to cover (and the practice of covering it). We might imagine that it could restore some of that bounding capacity, since the innate design is there for their magnificent rebounding power.

We have that innate capacity in our tissues, too. It is a deep issue. It takes time to restore, however, it doesn't necessarily take much *at a time!* It is more about persistence and consistency if we are to rediscover access to the range of movements we are designed for. The dose and degree matters – it can be 'a little bit over time' to restore the spring loading. Indeed, it is more about removing what doesn't work and improving what does in short doses that re-establishes and eventually accumulates our confidence in the innate ability to bounce. Human bodies are designed to spring. It's a magical ingredient of the structure.

I taught restorative yoga to seniors for many years. It was mostly down to one or two classes per week of relatively slow, always subtle, movements with persistent care of feet and subtle spirals for the limbs and torso. There were three stories that came up frequently.

1. 'I seem to have a spring in my step',
2. 'I am walking better',

and the magic one:

3. 'I tripped over and thought 'oh no, this is it' but I bounced! I couldn't believe it. How did that happen?'

I remember Val, who was in her seventies, and Bill, who was in his eighties, at the time. Bill came back from a dog walk in the park, covered in mud because he'd 'gone flying' but realized nothing was damaged and walked back! God bless them!

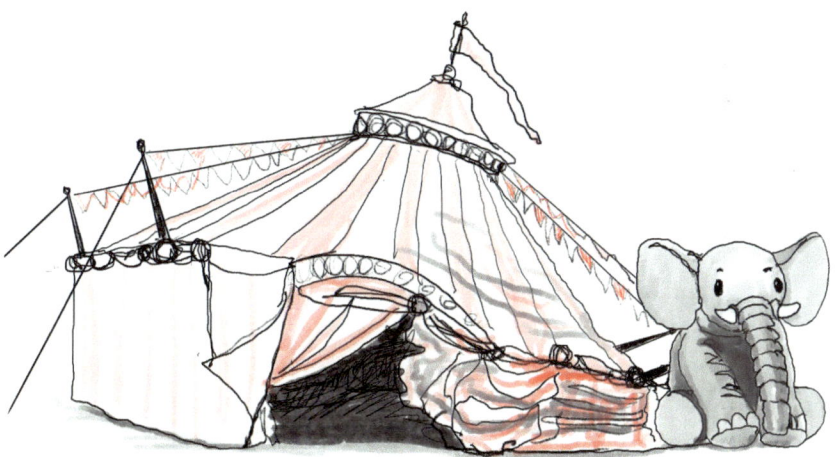

Figure 33 Sometimes an insult or injury to the body can seem like an 'elephant on the guy-wires' compromising the whole structure. It changes the tension–compression *result* by distorting and disorganizing the volume. A snapped Achilles tendon for example will compromise the structural integrity of the entire body and it will find itself unable to fill and move through space as it did before, until the structure is fully restored.

Many people are born with issues that prevent the full capacity others may have. Others may be injured and suffer changes to their movement range. Yet the structural integrity of contained tension and compression are still fundamental to their design. Every one of us has stored energy capacity. It is expressed by each of us uniquely, just as our bodies all look different, so the variations on how they contain and organize this capacity is different. It is invariably unique.

Essentially, fasciategrity honours the fundamental principle of how we self-organize as rounded forms, surrounded by gravity, bound together and able to bounce off the ground and bound to return to it. In other words, we are earthbound. Inside and out. Every part of us is designed with this 'spring loaded' built-in energy storage capacity. Just by breathing and swallowing food, we use it. Some people cannot lift off the ground, so their rebound capacity is restricted. We move to the next level of its expression, which is recoil. It becomes more subtle as we work through the five levels until we get to refine (see The Five Rs in Part 4). It is *always* relative.

Every strand of the body fabric, the tissue everyone is made of (at the microscopic level), is made of three triple-helical, spirally configured threads that form the weave of every body. It is something like three-ply rope, but so subtly and variously designed for the different functions the body incorporates, that it will take another book to explain! This fabric of fascia forms tubes and sheets with various names, from particular named vessels to sheaths and wrappings called aponeuroses, throughout the body. It is continuously holding, wrapping, and containing everything within us. We call it the 'fascial matrix' for want of a better term, and it is the foundation of how muscle fibrils within fibres, fibres within muscles, and muscles within muscle groups, form. Every strand of the fibre that muscle protein is contained in, is a triple-triple helix structurally. That is its forming pattern.

In fasciategrity, it is helpful to imagine that we are made of one muscle, pressed into place in hundreds of points around the body. They are all intimately connected to each other when you consider that the wrapping of all of the muscle protein becomes tendon; it isn't a separate add-on to the end of the muscle. When someone snaps an Achilles tendon, for example, it doesn't just locally disengage the calf muscle from the muscles and bones in the base of the foot, allowing them to limp home. The entire body is compromised, not just the 'back line' that Tom Myers made famous in Anatomy Trains™.

The Superficial Back Line theory shows the muscles of the back of the legs and torso in a continuum up to the cranium. Those muscles are not separate from the deeper ones they wrap, or the ones either side of them that live as neighbours. That line is 'cut out'. The whole body is brought down by such an injury (see Figure 33, how the insult 'the elephant' affects the whole structure), which is likely to be where its name came from – in battle, one arrow or blade to the Achilles tendon brought down the man. As a clearly visible and apparently relatively small point on the body, breaking that tendon makes it a point of high vulnerability.

It demonstrates well why the highly tensioned nature of this tendon as a continuity plays such a crucial role in the catapult-type recoil we rely on to walk and run. Think of kangaroos and we understand why some aspects of the fascia have the tensile strength of steel. Yet they rely on the counterbalance of compression resistance of the bones they enclose. Consider the size of a kangaroo's hind legs and you begin to see how these forces co-create the capacity to store energy when needed, fit for purpose. The kangaroo doesn't extricate bounce, or borrow it from a tree. It uses the ground as a temporary energy source and relies naturally on its own architecture to harness and translate this magical resource in a force transmission process over the territory it travels on. (See Part 4, Rebound.)

The fabric of the myofascia is within and around every aspect of the micro-to-macroscopic muscle, joining it continuously to the next muscle along (in all directions). You could imagine a string of sausages to help 'see' how the pocket that the meat is packed into is then twisted and spiralled between each filled pocket. Weaving many such strands together, without disconnecting them, would give you the pattern of the myofascia on all scales. That is within the fibrils, the fibrils to the fibres, the fibres to the muscle forms, the muscle forms to the muscle groups, and the groups to the whole body. None are disconnected from any other – top to toe and inside to skin.

Every myofascial continuity (in a sense, there is only one) is formed in ways that recoil by the nature of its organization. The bones tension the surrounding tissues (think of the spokes of the umbrella). The tissues compress the bones (think of the fabric of the umbrella) *but* they also tension and compress within themselves. It is a most marvellous phenomenon. Each bone and each tissue is, in and of itself, a tension–compression (or living tensegrity) architecture. It is the basic forming principle. It is the foundation of living soft matter. It is the 'Deus ex machina' of Blechschmidt's embryo.[8] There is no machine – it's your living fabric taking shape and holding itself in whatever shape it's in, to express itself as you in the round.

8   Blechschmidt, E. (2004) *The Ontogenetic Basis of Human Anatomy: A Biodynamic Approach to Development from Conception to Adulthood.* Ed. and trans. B. Freeman. Berkeley, CA: North Atlantic Books.

THE MAGIC OF ROUND THINGS

Consider every cell of us is somewhat like a water balloon. The water inside the balloon is reaching out, while the skin of the balloon is pushing in. That relationship between the internal material and the external skin is a similar balance of forces as the fabric of the umbrella and the spokes of the bicycle wheel. They are co-creative, mutual forces. The key to understanding fasciategrity is that every single part of you is combining these two forces all the time. What's more, that co-creation is the third force. The pushing out is the water (which is the compression aspect), the pushing in is the skin (the tensional aspect). One force *force-transmits* the other force, into animation. The compression creates the tension, and the tension creates the compression and, together, they unite into a tension–compression architecture. All three form the holy trinity of living form.

WHY SHOULD ANYONE CARE?

It is the basis of living structure and without it, bodies would deflate like a pierced balloon, or a discarded wetsuit when it's been peeled off the skin. None of us can peel off the skin, it is literally holding us together, held out by that which is inside, *keeping it tensioned,* and that which (at the same time) *the skin is keeping compressed.*

The body's internal organs can fold and unfold, but they don't flat pack! They are held in place by that which is keeping them compressed: the skin at the outermost structure and the gravity of the planet that is holding it in place. Everyone is surrounded by gravity, 24/7 in 360 degrees of roundness, all the time. It took nine months of growing (in a gravity-free environment) as a tension–compression architecture, contained by another tension–compression architecture, inside an outer skin called a womb. Every body (yours, mine, theirs) expanded inside a space that expanded to contain you, me, and them, as it held us in and we pushed ourselves out. That womb then restored itself, transformed back (somewhat as an umbrella folds away), ready for the next rainstorm, to be opened again. (See Part 4, Recoil.)

You literally grew yourself into the spring-loaded folds you call joints, enclosed in something that gently and appropriately wrapped and pressed you from the outside in, so you could grow from the inside out.

It's a law of nature and her exquisite co-creative forces that made you so that you could coil and spring. You are a recoiling structure designed to rebound and release and restore your shape and refine it. We can call it a spring in our step, or the ability to push a door open or turn the pages of a book or sit down without taking the shape of the chair. Even standing up from sitting down (and vice versa) is an example of our stored energy capacity, if we know how to fund those movements and naturally replenish them.

That innate recoil capacity is in everyone; it is how we move a finger or bat an eyelid. The lid doesn't drop and stop. It springs open and closed. The bladder doesn't empty once and deflate, it refills. So do the lungs. So does the heart. It isn't so much of a pump as an exquisitely spiralled, self-organized tubular wrapping system. It fills (sucks) and empties (spurts) blood around the body through its spiral nature.[9,10] It is more like a cloth that squeezes out and sucks in the fluid it organizes around the body, all in an enclosed system of exquisitely designed soft-matter architecture. The mama doesn't give birth and accommodate a uterus the size of twins or triplets for the rest of her life – the womb restores most of its shape for their siblings. We don't pick up a glass to drink and then destroy it by forming a fist that stays clenched ever after – we release the glass. Every move we make, from the breath to the rest, requires recoil and release. We have to be able to restore our balance, our fasciategrity, our structure. Then we can refine it.

That, right there, is free energy storage capacity. It is already in us – we just didn't call it that. I call it magic, myofascial magic, because we all have access to it, to a greater or lesser extent. We can all get more skilled, relative to our own age and stage of fitness, if only we know where to focus and how to fund this treasure we were born with (see Part 5). As movement teachers, we have the power to transform it for our clients, once we know how to spot the change that makes the difference for them. We can also use it for ourselves, patiently over time. It is an everyday resource.

We may not spend our lives focused on peak performance like an athlete or a member of the national ballet corps. However, we can use

9   Sharkey, J. (2021) 'Fascia and tensegrity: The quintessence of a unified systems conception.' *International Journal of Anatomy and Research* 9, 1.2, 7874–7880.
10   Torrent-Guasp, F., Buckberg, G. D., Clemente, C., Cox, J. L., Coghlan, H. C. and Gharib, M. (2001) 'The structure and function of the helical heart and its buttress wrapping. I. The normal macroscopic structure of the heart.' *Seminars in Thoracic Cardiovascular Surgery* 13, 4, 301–319.

our stored energy capacity so much more than most of us do because we don't realize we have it. It's free energy. It's there for us to store and restore once we know how it works. It is already in us. It isn't mythical, yet it is a little mystical, simply because the culture we learned in is framed in a mechanical metaphor. The wrong metaphor. The one that missed human nature as nature's human expression.

Delicious and nutritious movement relies on that magical source/ sauce from strong to subtle! In the next parts we will explore the main ingredients of our energy storage capacity through the five Rs. We go from reanimating the least to the most subtle and recognize what an incredible resource Mother Nature designed us to store within the structure of every single one of our trillions of cells, whichever system or structure they form into and integrate!

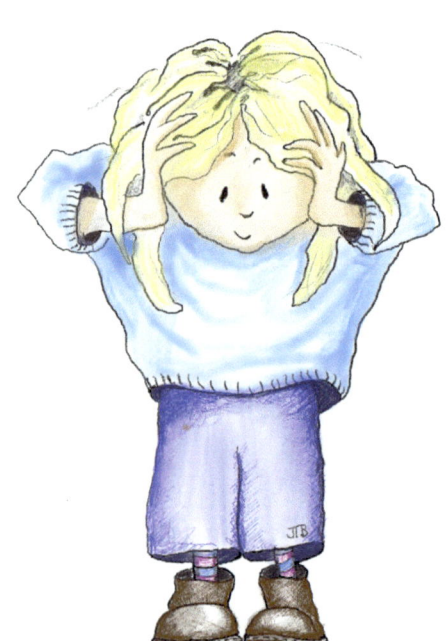

Figure 34

Adult human beings are considered to have 70 trillion cells – living, regenerating, and organizing their bodies into form. What does 70 trillion cells even mean?

There are considered to be in excess of 37 trillion human cells in our bodies. (Some sources cite more than 30 trillion bacteria in our body ecosystem, which is where the 70 trillion figure comes from.) Whatever the numbers, we represent a co-creative system. Even if we consider the general consensus, how much is 37 trillion? The point here is to get a sense of how extraordinarily huge that is as a number. It is hard to imagine, so let's put it in the context of time.

If we imagine a single second as 'one'.

A thousand seconds would be just over 16 minutes.

A week includes 604,800 seconds.

A 30-day month is 2,628,288 seconds. That is just over two and a half million seconds.

31.5 million seconds (approximately) represents a year.

A billion seconds is about 31 years and 8 months.

A trillion seconds is approximately 31,710 years. A trillion seconds ago, the Earth was in the grip of the Ice Age.

37 trillion seconds ago (using a trillion as 10^{12}) is 1.17 million years ago.

It's a lot; so huge it is hard to imagine. That many cells are renewing every day. That is, in and of itself, a wonderful mystery, one that is already part of your natural biomotional intelligence. Always moving. In motion while you are alive. With no mechanical parts. Every living cell. Each one a mini-me – of you!

SOMASENSE – THE INNER MUSIC

The second magical ingredient resides in the somatic senses or inner somasense. We can consider this our innate 'fascia feedback sensory awareness system' which is essentially a unique and personal resonance field. It is our inner music. Often, when we can hear it (which the practices in Part 5 are designed to promote), it offers us newfound congruency. There is an ability to express the being and the body together with more ease, effortlessness, and relaxation.

The previous section on structure considered human 'pre-tensioned architecture' which is a vital feature in the structure of many musical instruments. In this section let's consider an orchestra, with the variety of designs of the instruments in each section.

The string instruments, such as cellos and violins, include various shaped (hard-matter) boxes, with carefully placed and carved holes in them. Over those are tensioned strings. Even if you are considering an electronic instrument, like a guitar, note that the strings are under tension, very specifically tuned to make their optimum sounds. The wind instruments are tubular designs with plugs and pegs and keys opening and closing the holes. If the bagpipes or an accordion is added here, it expands the theme. The percussion section includes (and is not limited to) tensioned sheets or skins (such as diaphragms) across the hollow shapes of their main bodies, in various materials. Even in xylophones and triangles, the shapes of the different instruments and the related beaters bring about the *emergent properties* of different soundscapes. A piano mixes percussion and strings with keys, and all these variations allow for the incredible diversity and opportunity of making music. (There are many other instruments to be found around the world, but for the purposes of this conversation, we will stay with familiar classical categories. None are omitted from this metaphor.)

The human body incorporates all such shapes, in varying degrees. It could be argued that bodies are all made out of the same soft-matter material (fascia), expressing a variety of textures and densities (from strings and tubes to sheets and keys or plugs) making each person a living orchestra. The extent to which that transforms into an ability to live in harmony or play the symphony any one might be capable of, has to relate to both the instruments, the composition and the players. It is little wonder that music is played in 'movements' and the languages are so similar.

Music and the instruments that it includes (anything that makes a sound, really) provides yet another powerful metaphor that implies great possibility and scope regarding each person's sense of well-being and congruency. The tissue, everywhere in the body, is strung like an instrument. If it is possible to optimize the flexibility of the strings, the function of the keys, and the integration of the different aspects, then it is possible to recognize ourselves as the musicians and find our voice or favourite music.

As in the structure section (where we are the archer, the bow, and the arrow), we are the instrument, the music, and the musician. If each are resourced and we can become more sweetly tuned to our own sounds, then there is access to an inner sense, of the Wisdom Body, listening out for us (and listened for by us) every day. It allows us to perform a wider range, a more subtle repertoire, a more appropriate response to life happening.

This self-sense gives us moment-to-moment and movement-to-movement access to the spirit of us that animates our motives and guides our motion, emotion, and biomotional intelligence.

THE SPIRIT

There is always another turn in the road, another vista opening up, another awareness coming into view, a deeper level of loving and of commitment to the journey. After a while, you don't really want there to be an end, either, because the journey is so much fun.

(John-Roger, DSS)[11]

This is not about spirituality or a specific spiritual practice or the idea of any religion or personal preference. It refers to the spirit of the occasion, or the spirit that animates each soul, resident as it is, in its own soma. The aspect of 'being' that was separated from the body 400 years ago in the study of human anatomy is vividly present, nonetheless. It refers to the animation of individual expression.

Everybody expresses their spirit archetypally, in unique patterns of behaviour that combine as their natural 'hallmark'. This refers to something beyond the personality or the preferences; it speaks to the persona that shines through all of the aspects of human beingness. Each being has their own style, their own ways, their own journey and the gestures each one makes along that path are invariably unique to them and the occasion. That is what is true about time. There is only present to move in. Anything else is a report on the past or a hope or an intention for something yet to come. Beings live in bodies that are made of fascia and move in multiple ways, including (but not limited to) the myofascial matrix. A being can be moved, or moving, emotionally as readily as physically. That is a response with physical attributes, however it shares the responsiveness.

What is so fascinating about the fascial matrix, when it is respectfully considered as a process instead of a 'thing', is that it calls into

---

11   John-Roger, Doctor of Spiritual Science Program; MSIA, PTS Doctorate Studies, Peace Theological Seminary and College of Philosophy, CA, USA.

consideration the inner focus on what animates it, not just the outer focus on 'doing the right thing' or seeking external sanction or approval to do it. Human beings are kindred spirits, something everyone knows.

Fascia is not a 'thing' (a part of human being, or apart from it). John Sharkey considers it as a process and as a clinical anatomist, exercise physiologist, and manual therapist (a rare combination) his decades of work call for careful consideration.[12] As Sharkey and Flannigan concluded, 'Fascia is a seamless process giving continuity to the body from the superficial to the deepest organs, in a continuous network of tensional and compressional forces called mechanotransduction.'[13]

The spirit naturally accompanies every one of the gestures everyone makes and stores them in the tissue, responding accordingly. Fascia is effectively the instrument of sound (or resonance) in the human body. (Where else can resonance go, if the tissues are mostly made of one variation of fascia or another?) It is known to be the transmitter or conductor of light throughout the form largely based on the body as a bound water medium.[14] The scientific threads that form the background of all these enquiries are explored in more detail in another book. (The next book in this series is devoted to the subject of fasciategrity. It explains the role of fascia as a tensegrity-based tension–compression system in great detail, making sense of human architecture and how we move through time and take up space as we do so – under the structural system of all non-linear biologic forms.) Here the description of fascia is simply to honour that you, me, and they are unique. The gestures each of you, we, and they make are, too. That is the same respectfully honoured shape, regardless of what shape it is in. Regardless of what colour it is. Regardless of race, creed, colour, circumstance, condition, or environment *every* spirit animates the body it animates.

When structure, somasense, and spirit are congruent, they combine as a foundation of biomotional intelligence. They are all present in each person anyway. Knowing that, resourcing that, is when this magic can happen.

12   Sharkey, J. (2023) 'Fascia as a process.' https://myofascialmagic.com/post/fascia-as-a-process
13   Sharkey and Flannigan, 'Towards a paramedical interdisciplinary definition of fascia supporting practitioners offering fascia-focused therapies.'
14   Cifra M. and Pospíšil, P. (2014) 'Ultra-weak photon emission from biological samples: definition, mechanisms, properties, detection and applications.' *Journal of Photochemistry and Photobiology B: Biology 139*, 2–10.

Part 4

THE FIVE Rs

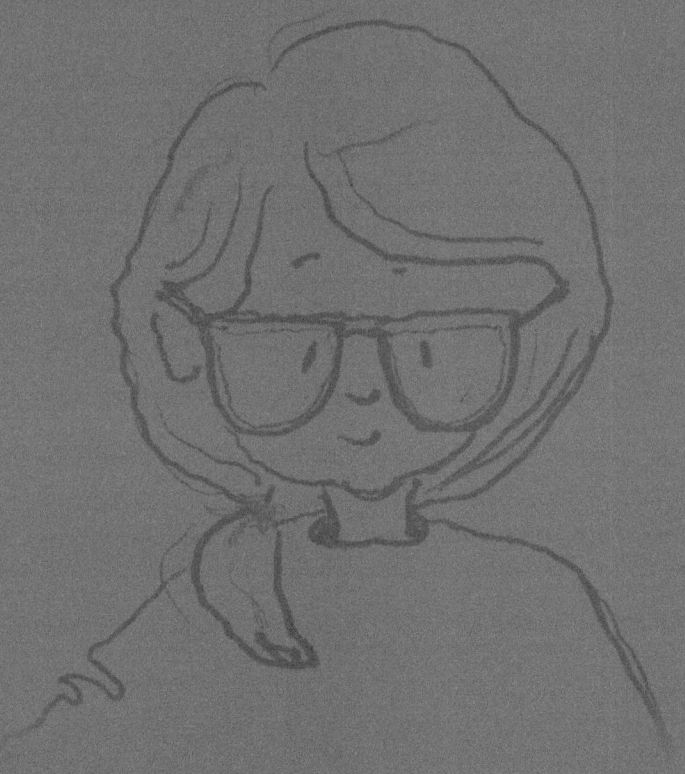

Overview and contributor chapters

FIVE Rs OVERVIEW

1. Rebound: when we spring off the ground print and leave the ground.
2. Recoil: when we stay within the ground print to build momentum.
3. Release: when we fold and unfold with appropriate constraint and ease.
4. Restore: when we replenish free energy storage capacity (elasticity).
5. Refine: when we finesse the potential to store and use free energy.

1. REBOUND

This is about moving over the ground and springing off it. Animals do it and so do we!

All the five Rs are interlinked, however, think 'bounce' when you are considering the definition of rebound. It refers to how human motion can optimize covering the ground with the contribution of rebound. Rebounding optimizes *energy storage capacity* and allows the body to travel through the air, as distinct from *along the ground, without losing touch with it*. It is visible in watching runners or athletes in any track and field event – recognizing the *lightness* with which they are able to bound over the surface.

Sprinters sometimes envisage the ground as a 'treadmill band', as if their feet can somehow 'roll it' underneath them while they travel over it. It links profoundly to the next R: recoil.

The challenge to the classical notions or biomechanical explanations for running are many and various. One example of research raises questions regarding tendon elasticity.[1] This research references an isolated aspect of the body, however, it is indicative of the twenty-first century approach to the essential foundation of rebound in the body-wide human tissue system.[2]

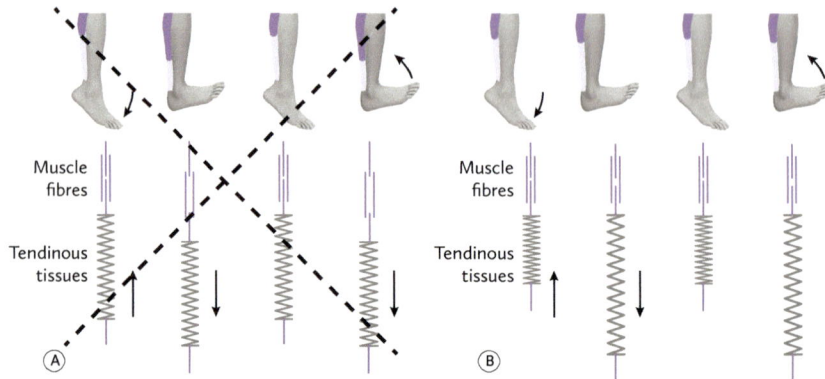

Figure 35 It was generally accepted that muscles change length and tendons remain the same – for example in the calf muscles and Achilles tendon in plantar and dorsi-flexion of the foot. Images of research by Kawakami and colleagues, show the cooperation of muscles and fascial tissues; their findings suggest the muscle length remains constant and the tendinous tissues change. Effectively this suggests that the muscles act more like brakes, while the tendinous tissues lengthen and shorten like springs. (A) is the classical assumption. (B) shows findings (after Kawakami).

Reproduced with permission from Art of Contemporary Yoga Ltd.

See Part 5 for rebound practice techniques designed to improve and resource rebound (see Part 5, Section 1).

2. RECOIL

In terms of activity, this is about *building momentum* within the 'ground print', and is less focused on springing off the ground, as spiralling from

1   Kawakami, Y., Muraoka, T., Ito, S., Kanehisa H. and Fukunaga, T. (2002) 'In vivo muscle fibre behaviour during counter-movement exercise in humans reveals a significant role for tendon elasticity.' *Journal of Physiology 540*, 635–646.
2   The discussion is taken further in Avison, *Yoga, Fascia, Anatomy and Movement*, Chapter 10: The Elastic Body.

it. It works at a slightly different frequency to rebound, within the same resonance field. Nevertheless, the balance and poise that all the techniques in the practices are designed to enhance is the intended result of focusing on this key aspect of myofascial magic. This facilitates a more subtle ability to respond that rebounding calls for, even though rebound and recoil support each other.

There is extensive research that changes all assumptions about how muscles activate motion via their attachments to the bones and the activating nerves, as the force distribution role of fascia is recognized and understood more fully. It is the context by which all these 'contents' of the body parts are supported. Fasciategrity explains this completely, making fuller sense of the 'magic' described in Part 3 of this book.[3]

Sprinters will use this recoil facility to spring from the blocks and 'catapult' themselves forward to prepare their rebounding over the track (see Rebound section for Dr Kelsick's view). In swimming, there is a completely different relationship to the watery environment, after the spring-loaded dive into the pool. There is not so much rebound as there is a dependency on good recoil through the water. Water does provide resistance that is minimized by shapeshifting (with contained spirals) in specific ways that optimize the ability to move *through* the water efficiently, rather than *over* it.

Recent research by Gatt et al. reports auxetic properties of not just the Achilles tendon, but in fact all tendons.[4] An unexpected mechanical property (called auxesis – which comes from the Greek meaning 'increase') shows that they get fatter rather than thinner when they are stretched, which is a first principle of fasciategrity – indeed all tensegrity structures – confirming their soft-matter, emergent properties.

(John Sharkey)[5]

As Dr Kirkness points out in her contribution to this part, recoil is innate to each body and part of how human beings become. Honouring it in the practice is providing an essential resource within. (See Part 5, Section 2.)

---

3   The next book in the series, *Fasciategrity in Motion,* is devoted to this aspect.
4   Gatt, R., Wood, M. V., Gatt, A., Zarb, F. *et al.* (2015) 'Negative Poisson's ratios in tendons: an unexpected mechanical response.' *Acta Biomaterialia* 24, 201–208.
5   Sharkey, J. (2019) Tensegrity Influenced Dissection Programme, Centre for Anatomy and Human Identification, School of Life Sciences, University of Dundee, Scotland.

3. RELEASE

Release focuses on changing the morphology of the tissues *appropriately* to the occasion and the person moving. Release can be facilitated through practitioner intervention and also 'self-release' using balls, rollers, etc. This has to be done carefully and thoughtfully, though. Simply 'whaling away' on tissue can distort it inappropriately, so it is necessary to be discerning about what is actually meant by the phrase 'myofascial release'. Release techniques can certainly help to free adhesion and *inappropriate* 'stiffness' or excessive strain, brought about by spasm or post injury and/or scarring or insult. However, it is also a phrase that can give rise to numerous misunderstandings. The term 'release' (much like the words 'stretching' and 'stiffness') can be misconstrued. They need a certain 'reset' in the light of twenty-first century anatomy. John Sharkey elaborates on these points in the contributory piece in this section.

When considering release, remember that 'insufficient stiffness' can do the opposite to optimizing energy storage capacity. In hypermobile tissues, for example, that can have the reverse effect of 'relief' and cause the tissues to leak energy rather than store it. Laxity can influence recoil and rebound in an undesirable way. As such, the techniques in the practical part under this section are designed to optimize the spring-loaded release principle (that is built into the body architecture) to balance tension and compression phase changes throughout the tissues. Essentially, it serves to 'release suboptimal patterns' through the *way* we move. (See Part 5, Section 3.)

4. RESTORE

This is about replenishing our energy stores so the capacity is restored. It is designed to promote recovery and deepen the reserves and resources available to the body, for all the five Rs. All of them can be depleted if there is insufficient consideration for this essential aspect of the fascia and myofascial matrix-in-motion.

In my experience, it is often the most overlooked of the five Rs. I am frequently faced with the issues and consequences of insufficient intervals between training or events and pushing beyond limits (particularly in athletes), as if that is a desired benefit. Getting this balance right is one of the richest sources of improving performance and removing pain. Often, I find my clients are suffering with unnecessary aches and strains, derived from low doses of 'restore and replenish' and high doses of 'over-training'.

This issue doesn't necessarily require clients to change what they are doing as much as shift the emphasis and balance *between* occasions and intensity and adjust the intervals between sessions, over a given time period. It is like listening to music. You would not enjoy any symphony if the orchestra did not 'play the pauses' or if it was all at one volume. The body is an instrument. Perhaps it would be more accurate to say, in essence, it is an orchestration of many different kinds of instruments. Our movement patterns can be considered our 'signature tunes' – and practice improves them – *if* we learn to restore and replenish the structural balance. All musicians have to rest, practice, and play around in order to perform well at their peak.

Key timing for restorative benefit is 45 minutes on and 15 minutes off, within the hour. Given the baseline, peak performance beyond that optimizes from a 30-hour interval between sessions for collagen synthesis.[6,7]

In the graph shown in Figure 36, optimum collagen synthesis occurs in approximately 30-hour intervals between training sessions. This allows the tissues of the matrix to recover hydration and recoil facility. That provides the release in the sense of the bow and arrow or catapult (discussed in Part 3) which then facilitates the restoring of free energy storage capacity. Essentially, this serves to 'restore optimal patterns' through the way we move. (See Part 5, Section 4 for the practice.)

6   The 'baseline' refers to whatever movement someone does on a daily basis. If the baseline is a sedentary practice, then all movements are above it. If the baseline is a daily dog walk, a daily swim, or a job that requires intensive movements (rather than sitting at a desk) then that can be considered the baseline. The preferred practice is then added to that, with optimum timing intervals. Elite athletics would include a low intensity baseline training and an optimal interval between those, taking into consideration that any event or peak performance would be considered optimized by the intervals in the graph in Figure 36.

7   Avison, *Yoga, Fascia, Anatomy and Movement*, Part 3.

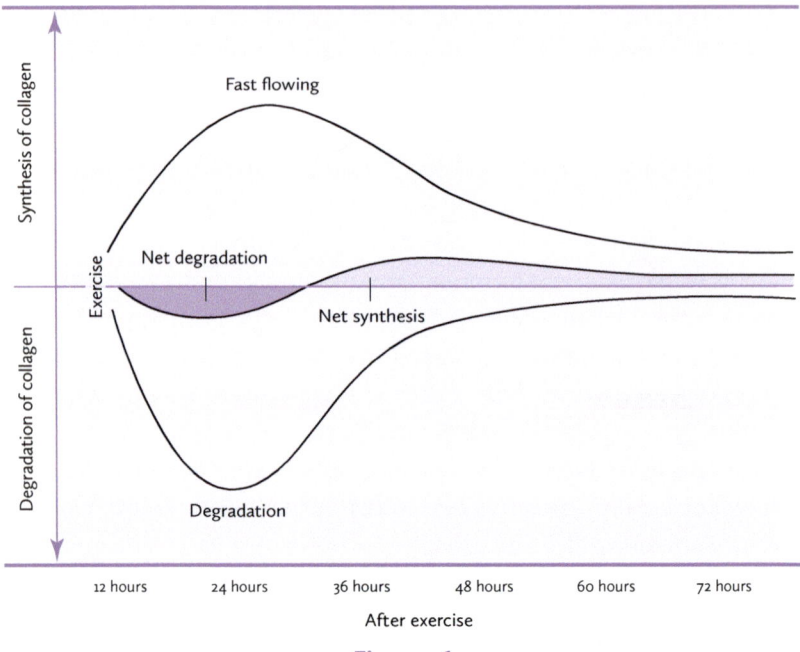

Figure 36

Reproduced with permission from Art of Contemporary Yoga Ltd.

5. REFINE

This is about refining our movements and working with micro-movements in a subtle and focused way. With no specific goal in mind (in terms of performance), these (like all the exercises) are designed to promote longevity, balance, spring, and self-confidence. Refining movements is to ensure that small, everyday issues like getting up and down stairs, carrying shopping, lifting children, reaching and bending down to do simple things, is effortless and happens without difficulty.

One of the major values in small, subtle, incremental movements is the cumulative effect they can have over time. These have a profound impact on our overall 'resting tone' and biomotional integrity. They are not quick-fix remedies. They are valuable resources for joining the dots of our specific training sessions (i.e., yoga, Pilates, personal training, gym sessions, martial arts, exercise class, running, etc.) with everyday use of myofascial movement pattern enhancers.

If we repeatedly engage in detrimental patterns (even unknowingly), they accumulate until a shape change shifts the overall posture profile. If, however, the same method is used to repeat *useful* patterns, the same effect accumulates, but one that might be more valuable, more 'proprioceptively optimal', or 'biomotionally intelligent' for our optimum shape and movement signature. It simply has us feel better!

Once you recognize it is part of the movement story *over time* of the fascia (our tissue of temporality), you can immediately set up small movement intervals that optimize useful cumulative changes. They can become the baseline practice. (See Restore section for more detail.)

To enhance each one of these five Rs there are the following resources:

- A section devoted to each one with a contribution from a key protagonist in the field of movement
  - Rebound – contribution by Dr Wilbour Kelsick, chiropractor, elite athletic coach
  - Recoil – contribution by Dr Karen Kirkness, clinical anatomist, yoga teacher
  - Release – contribution by John Sharkey, clinical anatomist, exercise physiologist
  - Restore – contribution by Helen Eadie, advanced yoga practitioner
  - Refine – contribution by Paul Thornley, Pilates instructor trainer, martial arts
- A practical training with illustrated sequences
- A practical course with live online coaching support here: https://myofascialmagic.com
- A deeper conversation (with references and bibliography) and a wider context for all the details touched on here in *Yoga, Fascia, Anatomy and Movement*[8]
- Podcast with lots of interviews with protagonists in the field and a variety of resources about Fascia. https://www.youtube.com/playlist?list=PL3NboJCvJRHImZG3-gLtJ3FaKXMeVp7UG

---

8 Avison, *Yoga, Fascia, Anatomy and Movement*.

Rebound

Dr Joanne Avison and Dr Wilbour Kelsick, with kind permission

REBOUND: THE FIRST R

When I was a kid in junior school, around eight to ten years old, we had 'play time' or 'break' when we were out in the playground together. One of the games we loved was called 'elastics'. It allowed us to play in a small group, to challenge ourselves and each other and it didn't take up as much space as skipping ropes, which tended to be relegated to P.E. class time.

Elastics was a girl's game! I'm not saying it should have been, but where I went to school, in the 1960s, that's what the girls did, while the boys generally preferred ball games in break time. Most of us had begged our mothers to buy a card of ordinary elastic tape, about 5 mm wide and tied the ends together in a knot, so that two of us could stand in the loop and hold it in a rectangle of about a metre long by looping it around our ankles and standing opposite each other with our feet hip-width apart. (We worked in feet and inches back then, but it looked something like that shown in Figure 37, with someone acting as a stand at each end of the rectangle.)

The point was that there was ample space for a third person to jump and step and 'do the moves' that went with playing elastics. The game was raised by literally 'raising the elastic loop' from ankles up to calves and eventually to knees, so the person jumping on and off the elastic bands, turning in the air, landing on the bands or crossing the elastics and releasing them, had to jump higher to clear them. When the jumper put one foot wrong (they didn't clear the elastic, or they missed stepping on it accurately for the move), it was the next person's turn. The player then took the place of one of the stands, and so it rotated. We played this jumping game between us for hours on end and we loved it. If there were more than three of us, but fewer than six, we simply formed a queue and carried on rotating. Everyone had their turn!

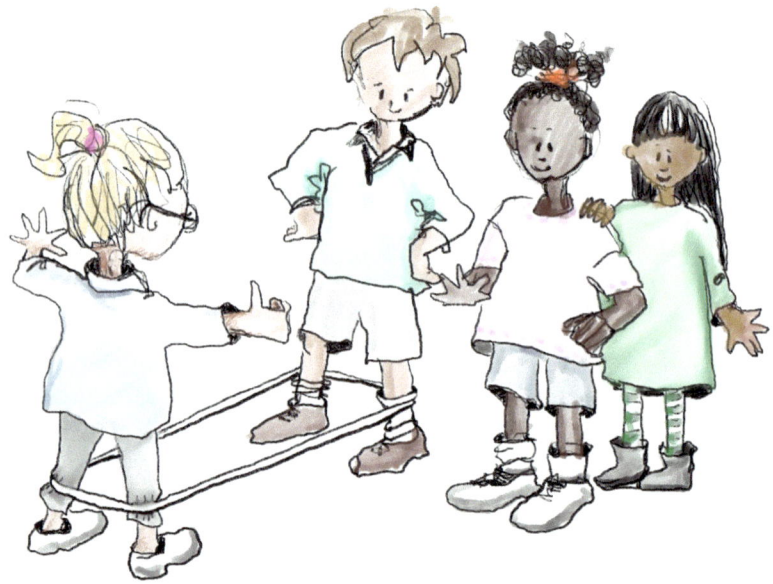

Figure 37

Somehow the competition element was designed to raise everyone's game and help each other to get better coordinated and more able to do 'fancy moves'. It really wasn't about beating anyone, rather it was to encourage and (without realizing it) teach ourselves to rebound and animate our feet and have a great time without going very far, in the breaks. We had no clue how valuable this self-organized training was for us. In those days, running was something you did for pleasure, a by-product of playing beach ball or tag or kicking a ball around; it hadn't reached the status it has today as a performance programme gauge or an elite athletics programme. We played elastics for fun, long before anyone had a clue that elastic rebound is part of the human body's basic genius.

One of my dearest colleagues, Dr Wilbour Kelsick, coaches in running, hurdling, and track and field with Olympic athletes. He treats their injuries, too, so we often chat about the value of training this essential aspect of myofascial magic. That is the first R, which is rebound.

I have no doubt that now, some 50 plus years later, 'elastics' could be banned for health and safety reasons. What we are saying here is that the fun and the frivolousness was a fabulous contribution to our fascia feedback systems. Little did we know it then, but we were training our 'rebound' faculty deep into our growing tissues. Moreover, we were having a great time doing it, as a by-product of playing together. This tissue of proprioception *knows* when it is enjoying itself. Between the parallel lines of light elastic tape, we were learning to spring load our tissues and coordinate their neuromyofascial magic as a deep resource throughout our non-linear forms. We were also learning how to turn ourselves in the air and spring *off* the ground as well as spring *onto* or *over* it.

We were recruiting a natural spring in our step, the ability to bounce up from a chair. It seemed to be synonymous with the enthusiasm to raise a hand in class and when a teacher asked us to do something, several of our hands would spring up begging to be chosen, just for the sake of participating. Somehow, the beauty of playful rebound went much more than skin deep. It gave us a relationship with anything we stood or sat on, and a readiness to bounce off it and bounce back on to it. It gave us a kind of light heartedness in far more than physical terms. Today I would say we were enjoying our natural *biomotional intelligence.* It was somehow part of how we could *be*, as well as what we could *do*.

We didn't dump our bodies into slumping. We sat still for 30 minutes in class lessons under duress, waiting for the bell to go so that we could get moving again! It was as much enthusiasm as restlessness – something in us couldn't wait for playtime when we could see if the next level of elastics was achievable. I imagine it is a soft introduction to things like Parkour today. At the time, it was sociable and delightful playfulness. To us, it was more like dancing. What we knew (whether or not we could have told you at the time) was when we were doing well, we were not only in the zone, but we were also in rhythm. It felt as if that rhythm was in our bones, and we loved it.

Rhythm could almost be the foundation of every one of the five Rs. It is the fundamental key to this one, rebound, because it helps us to syncopate our natural ability to bounce. We humans are on the other end of the spectrum to trees in terms of mobility. They live and grow rooted to the ground, and so do we. However, we get to take the ground with us as we move over it. It serves us just as intently, storing energy for us to restore with every step. However, the biomechanical mythology around walking and running gait is as tricky a metaphor applied to human running as it is to any other movement. There are other factors we have to bring in and, in this section, Wilbour's contribution describes how rhythm and rebound form the foundation of elite track and field athletics.

We keep repeating this: we are not machines. One of the reasons engineers have found it so extremely difficult to create a robot that can walk (let alone run or hurdle like an athlete) is that the mechanics that explain human walking are insufficient at best and, at worst, redundant.

This is not meant to be disrespectful, it is just not how elite athletes get gold medals. It's a practical matter, with real life variables and variety and those results don't come from biomechanical laws. They come from people. I have colleagues who have written books about the mechanics of walking gait, and they remind me of the scholars in the sixteenth century who designed complex mathematical theories about how planets moved in relation to the earth. Back in the sixteenth century, the Earth was considered to be The [most important] Planet, the celestial body at the centre of the galaxy. These scholars designed complex theories of 'epicycles' to explain how the pattern of each planetary orbit must operate in relationship to the Earth, in an Earth-centred (geocentric) basis of studying the movement of the spheres.

Despite their scholastic endeavours (or individual brilliance), the moment Galileo (1564–1638, a contemporary of Descartes and alive almost a century before Sir Isaac Newton) upheld Copernicus' theory that the sun was at the centre of our galaxy, it made all their scholarly theories redundant. They didn't relinquish them lightly – Galileo was placed under house arrest for his heretical views. It was one thing to suggest that Divine Man could be dissected, saved by the condition that the divine aspect guarding the soul and spirit remain under the jurisdiction of the Church. It was quite another suggesting that Earth, the *home* of Divine Man, was *not* at the centre of the Heavenly Galaxy. It was unthinkable at the time that God would place Hu-man anywhere other than front and centre in any aspect of education. It didn't follow religious principles which were guardian at the gate of humanity, particularly in Galileo's time and culture.

Galileo (who studied medicine, philosophy, and mathematics at the University of Pisa and became Professor of Mathematics in 1592) didn't let house arrest stop him. He published work to demonstrate that *every mathematical and geometrical theory simplified* and made perfect sense if the sun was at the centre of the galactic orbits and relationships. He could demonstrate that the fundamental geometry of every moving sphere in the galaxy was universal if a heliocentric foundation was established. There was no need to discuss epicycles; they became redundant. All the planets honoured the same 'centre' in their own unique ratios and relationships to the sun. Earth was relegated to the status of 'another planet' and a paradigm shift in understanding facilitated the amazing achievements of space exploration we enjoy in the modern era. At the time, it wasn't just wrong, it was *unthinkable*, regardless of how it transformed understanding and progressed education centuries later. People get very attached to history, and once it becomes legend, we forget it was a metaphor in the first place.

It is my personal belief that something similar is taking place in understanding the human body, resonant as it has to be with the celestial bodies, as nature's forms. We 'think' we are brain-centred and focus our understanding on the logical deductions of biomechanics. The shift in understanding fascia takes us back to the beginning, the embryonic genesis of each and every one of us. We are heart-centred, and the growing cardiac cells bring syncopation to the forming of the brain and spinal structure and shaping of the whole body's fascial architecture and orchestration. We rely on rhythm at a level so innate to our beingness that the sacred sound of our heart beating is taken for granted, unless it's being measured to check our blood pressure or fitness. Listen for a moment; it is your body's most sacred sound. It is life-force itself resonating through you.

What does a heliocentric galaxy have to do with rebounding? Well, a great deal. If we consider that the 'joints' in the original authorship of Aristotle's *De Motu Animalium* were described as 'resting points', and that a body is anything but a machine, then a lot of 'biomechanical gait analysis' becomes as redundant as the epicycles describing planetary movement around the Earth. The sun is at the centre. No standardized epicycles required. The heart is at our centre, no standardized gait analysis required.

If the so-called joints of the toes, the ball of the foot, the heel, the knee, and the hip and so on, are the resting points – we might consider them folds in the body continuity of our matrix. Each fold springs back (rebounds) and lands at a different frequency and resonates forces through the body, in feedback from the ground, uniquely for the task in hand and the person doing the rebounding. Gait analysis becomes a sensory feedback issue between coach and athlete at the time. The focus is to train rebound into their tissues as a facility! One form, or feature, or fascial organization does not fit all. *Ever*. The following piece from

Dr Kelsick reiterates this holistic, body-wide view of the forces that the body negotiates and how they organize through the entire structure.

1. Finding rhythm

One of the keys that Wilbour conveys at length to his athletes, without exception, is the importance of 'finding their rhythm'. Every one of them is in a unique relationship to the track depending on their hydration, their body weight/mass, their mood, and readiness on the day. He can only optimize all the conditions; he can't authorize or control a standard response as if it is a mechanical result of each condition in place. No one has that kind of control. What he can do, is reassure himself and his athlete that they have built-in optimization for rebound into the tissues. That's the focus of their pre-habilitation training. That way, the instinctive default for that athlete, the common denominator of their focus is optimum rebound facility, whatever that is for them. This will come into all the points following and act as their inner library of default resources.

Wilbour writes:

> *Human gait and locomotion are governed by a complex rhythmic communication interaction between the lower extremity, pelvis, trunk–neck–head and upper extremity. In other words; the coordinated whole. It's a true example of perpetual exchange of stored energy in a closed biological system.*

2. Amplitude

Once the rhythm is found and established over a particular running or jumping distance (and/or intervals of hurdles, for example) then the focus is on timing and amplitude. The ligamentous structures in the body, particularly in the lower extremities and the pelvis (sacro-iliac joints, sacro-tuberous ligament, among others) are highly pre-tensioned and suitably stiffened with tremendous rebound and recoil capacity within the design. This facilitates stored energy capacity and appropriate release of energy, at the right time (see 1. Finding Rhythm). These and other ligaments and structures (not just those in the pelvis) offer the tensile strength of steel, according to Deane Juhan in *Job's Body* (see p. 83). The combined features of the lower girdle and limbs work in simultaneous harmony amplifying (and tuning) each other's production of energy regardless of which structure initiates the movement.

Wilbour gives us various examples of this as follows:

...in running, jumping, or hopping there is a journey, or an interactive series of pathways, of the ground forces from toes to head and through the entire body. In such activities, after the initial contact of the foot with the ground, there follows a sequence of counter movements. These allow for (or generate) the amplifying effect of ground reaction force (GRF) to move through the lower extremities to the pelvis, then into the spine and torso, through the trunk and upper body to the head. It could be argued that the movement is initiated from the head down, which animates the first foot placement, so it is a body-wide inclusive energy circuit-in-motion, wherever the analysis starts!

For jumping or hopping (as with walking and running), to be biologically efficient or biologically economical, the system must be suitably pre-tensioned. It is innate to the design organization of the architecture of the tissues. This pre-tension is augmented by using specific body postures and positions, by animating specific angles in training at ankle, knee, and hip for example. This trains the body to attain the right amplitude for bounding, hurdling, jumping, or hopping (which is what running really is). For example, dorsiflexion of the ankle joint (in the air) in preparing for a jump squat or bounding jump is an essential amplification for pre-tensioning that the athlete learns to perfect. In any of these body movement activities the features of timing and coordination are crucial in executing a smooth, rhythmic sequence that practices and promises efficient and effective outcomes.

Hurdling is a great activity to demonstrate whole-body rhythmic movements with timing, pre-tension and coordination at the heart. Hurdling is exaggerating what the body is designed to do in walking or running, when it includes stepping over obstacles. In hurdling the runner needs to 'set up', or prepare, the body posture before attempting to get over the hurdle.

This involves some pre-tension postures and stances and positions and force transmission techniques, so that the runner's relationship to the ground as they approach the hurdle is optimal (and at the right amplitude) for the leap. In hurdling, the timing of upper extremity action and lower extremity action has to be in perfect synchrony for efficient and effective execution over the hurdle. This then has to sequentially 'set up' the athlete for the next hurdle ahead. The upper and lower body and the limbs are not separate; they work simultaneously coordinating, but from contralateral spirals. The right lead leg moves and extends forward, and the left arm extends backward. The pelvis and trunk become the temporary centre of coordination. They act as the 'switching point' for that left–right coordination of upper and lower extremities while travelling the pelvis through the air, over the hurdle.

This contralateral spiral motion establishes the rhythm which is needed to set up the ground contact (GRF) by the lower extremity (foot) to propel the body upwards and forwards over the hurdle. This sets up the efficient rebound that must follow the leap-into-land prior to the next hurdle. It must do so with uninterrupted rhythm, so the body doesn't land and stop or decelerate. Essentially the body 'collects' the GRF in cyclical rhythm (at the right amplitude) to set up the next hurdle in a continuous repeatable rise-and-fall sequence.

Hurdling is one of those sporting activities which demonstrates that full body movement, dynamic postural pre-tension, force amplification, bio-elastic recoil, cyclical energy exchange, timing and coordination in the myofascial, neurofascial and osseofascial network work together throughout the human body. Rebounding is almost impossible to explain broken down into linear, biomechanical terms.

For the being doing the sport, it is often the ability to find their rhythm and amplify it appropriately, that gives them the mysterious keys to unlocking this demanding sport's highest rewards and seamless rebounding. (Not to mention the athlete's intention and determination and focus, which are all part of the living equation!)

3. Travelling the pelvis – the cyclical sequence

The next feature to consider (and needless to say, this all happens at once in elite training grounds) is how well and easily that athlete can 'travel the pelvis'. It is part of the rhythm and amplitude (see above) but merits a few comments of its own, from Wilbour:

Walking and running are the most natural and instinctive motional behaviours in human locomotion. They are the basis of how we humans survived from predators and fed ourselves. Both activities (walking and running) involve cyclical phases. However, there is a major difference in that walking has a double leg support phase which is not present in running. By contrast, running has a double leg floating phase (both legs off the ground) which is not present in walking. In both walking and running there is also the recovery leg which is the stance taken by the back leg which stores the rebound momentum in the ground contact cycle. When this is appropriately harnessed for that athlete, it allows the foot to clear any obstacle on the ground during forward propulsion which, in hurdling particularly and also running and jumping, is airborne. The pelvis is travelling through the air, not rolling along the track. It has to respond to GRF and float! This cyclical approach is a very important feature and characteristic of both quadrupeds and bipeds.

We even have to enter a new appreciation of human 'unipedal motion' when the body is rebounding into the air. Bear in mind that kangaroos and rabbits 'hop' on two legs. Human's hop on one leg and spend a part of every gait cycle on one leg. Hurdling is quite distinct from jumping and other track and field events like long jump (although that can include a kind of airborne running) and two-legged landing stances. They all require slight variations in how the pelvic travel is animated and sustained and how the rebound action integrates and transforms GRF appropriately. (It looks effortless in action!)

Wilbour adds:

Human locomotion and what is called 'ambulatory capacity' is designed as a perpetual gait system which allows the coordinated motion of the arms and legs, with the pelvis as a kind of transition zone, to act reciprocally storing potential energy and converting it to kinetic energy in the process.

Understanding how to translate that information into performance, takes care and practice as it is invariably unique to each athlete and each of their events. It is one thing to write a commentary and quite another, as a coach, to facilitate that ability in an athlete!

4. Centre of mass balance

This is another (not separate) aspect of this propulsion through the air. Both upper and lower girdles play a role. However, the general gait of humans is on the feet, rather than the hands, although we are able to use our whole bodies. Fasciategrity principles remind us that the torso is not carried along like a passenger on the legs, held together by the pelvis. If the stacked body of twentieth-century biomechanics were the case, gymnasts and high-jumpers would routinely lose their legs (or at least injure their spines) when they rely as heavily on their arms and shoulder girdles for propulsion over the ground (or with a pole to vault) as they need to do. The whole body is part of a tension–compression architecture that retains structural integrity in all positions in 360 degrees of motion by the living body structure.

The ground is used to *transfer* forces, usually referred to as ground reaction force or GRF. Those forces are transferred *through the form* and converted by the trained athlete into propulsion. At elite levels, this becomes very specifically controlled to reach their optimum goals and win medals.

Wilbour writes:

Generating, coordinating, and transferring energy from the GRF to the body system allows the athlete to move forward or hop, leap or propel themselves over obstacles. As the saying goes, 'What goes up must come down' and 'for every action there is an equal and opposite reaction'.

To put it simply, for efficient and effective human propulsion we need a sequence of rhythmic ups and downs of the pelvis, where the centre of mass (CM) is located in the body in upright motion, on track and field. We also need the CM to travel horizontally to cover the distance.

This marriage of ups and downs and horizontal translation of the CM is what leads to propulsion or the forward motion. This is true cycling of energies (potential and kinetic). The discussion is usually based on shifting the CM vertically and horizontally, however, what it actually results in is a sinusoidal wave pattern. As mentioned earlier, humans are non-linear biologic forms.

As a coach working with elite athletes, I have to view these pattern shifts and energy exchanges as if they are biological musical sheets; something like a repertoire of rhythms. That way, I can conduct all the different players towards their best, integrated performance! It cannot be fully expressed in reductionist terms of up and down and forward and back, simply because the body doesn't move that way! It rebounds and recoils, as we have shown, which is essentially more like a spiral sound wave.

Regarding the force action and reaction principle: in any locomotion or movement (walking, running, jumping) with ground contact, the GRF is dependent on the force applied through the foot. The greater the force of foot contact to the ground the greater the GRF to the body initiating movement. That means the harder or stronger you hit a drum or drag a bow across the strings of a string instrument, the louder the music in return. It affects the amplification directly. The next question arises from the kind of symphony that is being played on the occasion and the appropriate amplitude at a given time. To win an athletic event, the coach, the athlete, the team, the track, the training, and so on all play into conducting the whole symphony. It can all be perfect, but if the rhythm is out, it will show, and the result is unlikely to be a medal! Often, we use the rhythm as the guiding principle for the right sequence, amplitude, and balance throughout the symphony of an event. It is a question of hitting the right note at the right tone and frequency, which will be unique depending on the athlete. Someone tall and slim can move as elegantly and effortlessly as another athlete with a completely different physique. It is about the individual being in tune and essentially in rhythm with the task in hand.

5. All the Rs

Wilbour summarizes his points this way:

Human locomotion has always been at the foundation of our survival as a species. It is essential to our existence in terms of nourishment and escaping predators. In the modern era we have developed our understanding of locomotion and many more people enjoy the elite levels of specialist performance in all sports and activities. Walking, running, jumping are all forms of locomotion and to varying degrees use the same principles as elite performance. They all rely on rebound as part of the facility. Behind rebound, the secret is often found in rhythm! Rhythm is unique to everyone.

Rebound is based in 'stored energy capacity' which is the foundation of the true meaning of elasticity. It isn't about how far you can stretch an elastic band, like the 'elastics' we used as children, that after our game scrunched easily into our pockets. In technical terms of elite athletics (the extreme level of performance) it is essential that human architecture is suitably pre-tensioned and stiff enough to rebound naturally, with maximum capacity to travel through the air and transmit rebound forces through the tissues. (Remember that steel has higher elasticity than rubber in the true sense of the word, because its stored energy capacity has greater rebound facility.)

The aim is to minimize energy expenditure and allow for effective execution of these modes of movement which human evolution has allowed us to achieve. Human or biological locomotion is a whole body/organism event and is not only dependent on any one body part. Several factors contribute to the entire body's ability to execute movement. The five Rs of rebound, recoil, release, restore and refine, take a holistic approach, based on the human body's innate recoil capacity and ability to exhibit pre-tension of tissues (we are formed as a pre-tensioned, or pre-stiffened, architecture). This permits the force amplification needed to perform at elite levels. All such tissues, however, have to practice (through appropriate repetition and training) the coordination and timing to find their own unique rhythm in the context of the constraints of their chosen sport, to make it look so supremely effortless. This in turn facilitates efficient energy generation and transfer, which allows the airborne body to travel, using the ground lightly beneath the feet, when needed, almost like a treadmill.

Wilbour adds:

Understanding or viewing the body as a truly integrated and self-perpetuating, non-linear biologic, dynamic system provides new insights into how we discover and diminish dysfunction and injury, and manage and promote solutions to create near-optimum function in the system. Efficiency in rebound is often the result of a deeply established rhythm that the athlete has learned to dial up and down and modify or amplify accordingly, whatever their best event.

Recoil

Dr Karen Kirkness

To have a body is to change its shape regularly and, more often than not, unconsciously. Being complex and multicellular means continuously shapeshifting as the dance of life wiggles its way from diapers to dust. This dance is more than multi-stable, it can be omni-stable – in the sense that by way of homeostasis, the body is always and everywhere seeking stability and normally manages to do so even when the individual parts are compromised.

The body is inherently coiled. Stability is maintained in the helical coil of tissue from the macro to the micro level. The rhythm of the seeking-but-never-owning-stability dance can be understood as tissue continuously responding to forces, complying as needed, and then coming back to the coil. The message contained within this piece is a call to action for women of all ages to prioritize recoil, that is, to embrace and nurture your strength.

Earlier in life, recoil is largely built in. One potent example of this propensity for recoil can be observed in the compliance/recoil of the phenotypically female body. In rhythm with the lunar cycle, typically female hormonal cascades may result in fertility and, eventually, pregnancy. The pregnant uterus becomes quiescent, the ultimately compliant hollow organ that continues growing to accommodate the developing neonate. And then, one fine day, that quiet compliance shifts to the polar opposite: activity, power, and...push.

The womb, from necessarily expansive to legendarily contractile, is nothing short of marvellous in its de-coil to recoil capacity. It experiences a 20-fold increase in its weight, from 50 to 1000 grams; a 1000-fold increase in its volume, from 4 to 4000 ml; and a 10-fold increase in circulation from 50 to 500 ml of blood per minute. The shape and location of the uterus, strictly a pelvic organ until 12 weeks, is fundamentally transformed as it shifts from elongated to oval to round by 12 weeks, then becoming decidedly abdominal as it displaces the majority of mama's viscera. The uterus returns through oval to elongated at term, well positioned for the slow oxytocin-led explosion to come. This profound expansion and associated shift in positioning could be likened to the moments before a powerful whipcrack, where the material gathers her potential energy in preparation for the almighty kinetic reflex.

Puerperium, from puer ('child') + pariō ('to bring forth, bear') is defined as the time from the birth of the placenta through the first approximately six weeks postpartum. Puerperium is very much the period of maternal recoil, helical on every level, beautifully illustrated in the spiral arteries 'screwing shut' to mechanically cauterize the maternal blood supply following labour. Blood vessels are intertwined by cross-ply myometrial fibres, an array of helical filaments tapering into ligaments we know by name: ovarian, cardinal, round, and uterosacral, as well as the uterine tubes. The double spiral arrangement of myometrial fibres investing the uterus allow for both its quiescent de-coiling and its powerful birthing recoil/reflex.

If the compliant phase of shape change, pregnancy, is characterized as gradually following the 40+ weeks of baby's growth and development, then sub-acute puerperium can be understood as the rapid 'bounce back' that happens over just six weeks. To get a sense of this, the pregnant uterus on its own (excluding baby, placenta, and fluids) at full term weighs approximately 1000 grams. After six weeks postpartum, the uterus returns to its normal 50–100 grams.

Oh – but ask any new mother how her body is feeling just six weeks after giving birth and one word you aren't likely to hear often is 'normal'. With baby and placenta expelled from her body, it isn't only the female reproductive tract that begins the recoil back to the prepregnant state, but the very fabric of the mother's being that experiences recoil after withstanding the limits of her compliance. Each holon – think 'mini system' – of mother's being has its own rate of rebound.

After six weeks, her uterus might weigh nearly the same as it did before she got pregnant, but it wasn't just the uterus that grew to accommodate her baby! Her spirit, neuroendocrine rhythms, abdominal tissue, perineum, skeleton, including teeth, her eyes and hair, feet and face – every system from gross to subtle – all dance with the demands of the tiny human deployed within her. Each of these holons in her self-holarchy behave according to their own intrinsic viscoelastic time-scale, so the rate of recoil is different for each interacting system. These various rates of recoil encourage and inhibit in both direct and indirect ways, giving rise to the individual postpartum experience, different for every woman. Recoil is never a linear path, but a rhythmic waltz taking us forward one minute and backwards the next as we twirl around the dance floor of parenthood.

What is surprising for many women, speaking from personal experience here, is that the tiny human becomes no less demanding of the accommodating spirit once they have their feet on terra firma! Parenthood represents an extended, seemingly endless rhythm of expansion – patience, sleep deprivation, unconditional love – marked by contractile ruptures that heal in their own time. As the spirit de-coils and recoils to manage the new forces of each progressive stage of life, so too does the body's smart fabric.

Tissue is indeed some pretty intelligent stuff. It tells the story in its own terms: the helical coil of collagen is a tighter substrate in youth, becoming slighter and ever more brittle with the passing of years into senescence. The onset of increased oestrogen supports collagen through menarche, cultivating fertility and ushering a woman into her child-bearing years.

Pregnancy concocts a potent biochemical cocktail that, among much else, recalibrates the brain to love our offspring with supernatural intensity. What's more, that cocktail – specifically, relaxin – alters the very weave of mother's fascial tissue. Her tighter tissue springiness is loosened to accommodate the growing baby, then her ligamentous skeleton is unlocked to grant baby safe passage through her pelvic canal, which is extremely narrow compared with other species. Relaxin essentially denatures – de-coils – the collagenous tissue to make it more compliant, an effect also associated with low oestrogen. The decline of oestrogen is related to the surge of prolactin that hastens the onset of lactation and breastfeeding, another cascade of expansion/contraction, de-coil/recoil, that the nursing pair experience together.

Of course, what a woman needs to fully lean into that tissue recoil, to 'get her body back', is more oestrogen! But if she wishes for more oestrogen, whether to get her body back or to stimulate ovulation again in pursuit of her next wanted pregnancy, then she is committing to a fall in prolactin. That fall in prolactin means the end of the breastfeeding relationship with her current baby – a recoil conundrum for many older mothers who desperately wish to offer their baby extended nursing but who are also longing deeply for a second child before her store of eggs comes to a non-negotiable end.

The timing of recoil has much to answer for, and it so often expresses itself in rhythms. That postpartum decline in oestrogen that can interfere with tissue healing is a recurring theme,[9] one that all women will experience at some point if they live through the full arch of their female phenotype. Menopause is increasingly shown to elicit a return of pelvic floor dysfunction for many women as the collagen support of oestrogen dwindles.[10] What's more, women must expect to live more than a third of their lives in a post-menopausal state, which means managing life with low circulating levels of the oestrogen and progesterone that essentially baste younger bodies in collagen-supporting juice.

Elderly postmenopausal women are known to suffer disabilities related to sarcopenia, the age-related loss of muscle mass and strength – the anathema of recoil. As Hansen points out, 'Resistance training and dietary optimization can counteract or at least decelerate the degenerative ageing process, but lack of oestrogen in postmenopausal women may reduce their sensitivity to these anabolic stimuli and accelerate muscle loss.'[11]

It is well established that oestrogen is a significant factor influencing skeletal muscle protein turnover, but sex hormones seem to affect the biomedical properties of tendons and ligaments differentially, non-linearly. Hormone replacement therapy (HRT) plays an important role in managing the onset of wastage and promoting tissue integrity for longer. However, there are distinct differences in how endogenous (from within) and exogenous (from outside) chemicals factor into the complex biochemical cocktail that so fundamentally characterizes the experience of having a body.

So, it isn't a case of relying on HRT to simply bail us out of declining female hormones. I contend that managing an increasingly ageing

---

9   Albers, L., Garcia, J., Renfrew, M., McCandlish, R. and Elbourne, D. (1999) 'Distribution of genital tract trauma in childbirth and related postnatal pain.' *Birth* 26, 11–5.

10   Hansen, M. and Kjaer, M. (2014) 'Influence of sex and estrogen on musculotendinous protein turnover at rest and after exercise.' *Exercise and Sport Sciences Reviews 42*, 4, 183–192.

11   Hansen, M. (2018) 'Female hormones: do they influence muscle and tendon protein metabolism?' *The Proceedings of the Nutrition Society 77*, 1, 32–41.

population requires large-scale educational outreach. The more we know as women about our bodies, the more empowered we may feel to get – and remain – strong, the longer we may benefit from the recoil response of tissue. Of course, the term 'strength' is not an easily measurable term. I'm using it here as more of a call to conversation. In the name of learning recoil, in the hope that we may become surprised by the impact of keeping our body work conversations centred around strength rather than defaulting to release, without recognizing the essential considerations of the 'other Rs' it works with in concert.

As older women, do we allow ourselves to be shepherded too early to the passive pasture? Living another one third of your life with lower levels of collagen-supporting elixir means shoring up that recoil with volition, attitude, and education. Changing the way we talk about training/healing tissue is an essential step forward for future generations of women who we need to remain strong enough in their wisest years to lead important conversations in an increasingly problematic world.

Release

John Sharkey, MSc

I believe that words are important. More than important, they are vital. While visual expressions are useful, words are the primary means by which we communicate, express our ideas, convey information, and share our thoughts, beliefs, and emotions with those around us. Our choice of words can significantly impact how our messages (i.e., what we truly mean to say) are perceived, understood, and interpreted. A general consensus among all scientists is that words and language provide a significant advantage in the development of human culture, cooperation, and cognition. So, if words are powerful, as I suggest they are, then taking time to choose your words with care helps to ensure we avoid the dreaded AI. No, not artificial intelligence but artificial information.

Lots of people use the term 'release' when talking about stiff muscle fibres, fascia, or connective tissue. It is important to note that the term is mostly used metaphorically and, therefore, it can be confusing as it does not always refer to a physical 'release' in the way one might think of it in everyday language. Instead, it seems that we use this descriptive word as a way of describing the intended outcome of certain therapeutic movement or manual modalities. The concept of 'release', in this context, is often associated with the idea of reducing tension, stiffness, adhesions, or restrictions that reside within our fascia or muscles. It is associated with the idea of something being pulled or torn apart, or perhaps made longer by being 'released'.

Fascia is a complex web of connective tissue that surrounds, penetrates, and interconnects all structures in the body, including muscles, bones, organs, and nerves. Myofascia is a specific type of fascia within the fascial matrix of the body, wrapping and penetrated by the muscle protein. It is believed that restrictions or adhesions and scar tissue within connective tissue, can develop due to trauma, insult to the fascia, inflammation, poor posture, or undue repetitive motions. These insults are thought to potentially cause discomfort, limited range of motion, or other issues. When therapists use the term 'release', they are generally referring to the application of techniques that aim to address such restrictions. The goal is to achieve a more pliable fascia, improve tissue mobility, and potentially alleviate discomfort and pain.

USING THE TERM 'INSULT' RATHER THAN 'INJURY'
A useful distinction can be made using the term 'insult' where there doesn't necessarily have to be an injury, as such. For example, inflammation due to bacteria or a virus could constitute an insult to the tissue. A fascial thickening can be the result of repetitive movements, or poor posture can result in what might be better referred to (particularly in the earliest stages) as an 'insult' rather than a specific injury. It is a less than optimal situation in the tissue and may refer to dehydration or minor compromise. It may lead to injury, and suggests something less obviously detrimental, or less impactful than an injury, although it may be undesirable.

On 11 February 1990, Nelson Mandela, the South African anti-apartheid revolutionary, political leader, and philanthropist, who became a symbol of resistance against racial oppression and a global advocate for justice and equality, was 'released' from prison. It is easy to appreciate and understand the word release in that context. However, is it possible to 'release' living connective tissue other than by cutting or pulling it apart during a surgical procedure? Are we truly *releasing* anything or is it simply a feeling we are trying to describe? Have we released the tissue, or the discomfort? It is worth considering because true tissue release has wider implications.

Let's explore the word release in more detail. The word 'release' is a verb that refers to the action of setting something free, granting freedom, or allowing something to be discharged, or let go, as was the situation with Nelson Mandela. 'Release' involves the act of freeing from confinement, control, restraint, or obligation. 'Release' can also pertain to emotions, tension, or information, implying a sense of liberation or *relief*.

In a broader sense, release can be the psychological outcome of letting go, for example letting go of sadness, fear, guilt, or anxiety, and that kind of cathartic release is to be encouraged and can have profound healing benefits in the right circumstances. Yet how can we explain 'release' specific to connective tissue? What would 'letting go' look like and how could we describe it and stay true to the reality of what takes place under the skin?

When a qualified therapist talks about 'releasing tension in a muscle', they could be referring to the process of *inhibiting* muscle fibres that were previously contracted and unsuitably tight. The outcome, under the appropriate treatment, is the *feeling of releasing pain and discomfort.* This appropriate inhibition can be achieved through the use of specialized neuromuscular or cognitive techniques. In the context of joint manipulation or mobilization, the term *release* could imply the reduction of restrictions or adhesions in a joint or associated tissues, resulting in improved range of motion and decreased discomfort. This is worth exploring, as it is an essential foundation to the notion of myofascial magic. It does not necessarily require surgical intervention to *literally* release adhesions, as if cutting them loose or free, in the example above. It does require the appropriate expertize to rehydrate and restore the natural motion of the tissues within the matrix – and it takes time to reorganize and adjust to.

In this context, such a release could cause micro tissue damage at the local point of adhesion, which can lead to a sense or feeling of soreness several hours later. This kind of release involves appropriately distinguishing, or 'separating apart' tissues that have adhered and lost their natural continuity and autonomous or seamless gliding within the matrix. These movements rely innately on appropriate tissue glide within the structures and between the neighbouring structures so that superficial tissue can move relative to deeper tissue. It may not be instant; however, it can greatly improve the site of the insult and redeem the situation to preserve the tissues and avoid injury.

This is sometimes referred to as, what appears to be, muscles 'free to contract and relax'. Care must be taken here as the idea of 'stiffness' or 'my muscle can't seem to relax' is misleading. Physiologically, muscles do not relax, ever. Regardless of how common this misconception may be, muscles *only* do one thing. They contract. Muscles are organized through a complex and intricate system of neurological inhibition. That means, effectively, that the balanced nervous system naturally inhibits the default contraction of the muscles, in the appropriate sequence or intervals. The muscles only contract. The nervous system integrates their inhibition. What appears to be superb muscular control in a dancer or gymnast (for example) is in fact superb neuromyofascial integration. Without it, movements can seem involuntary or uncoordinated. This is a supremely important aspect of the more subtle movements in this book, that are designed to help the body thrive and honour the intricacies of this foundation of human motion.

NEUROLOGICAL INHIBITION

From a neurological point of view, inhibition of muscle tissue involves a complex interplay of neurotransmitters, receptors, and neural pathways working together to reduce the excitability and activity of muscle fibres. The muscle fibres could be described as 'always switched on' if they can be. When the neurological inhibition works seamlessly to 'switch them off', while they maintain their structural organization, movement becomes subtle and seamlessly coordinated. This process is crucial for maintaining muscle tone, preventing excessive or unnecessary contractions, and allowing for controlled movements whatever movements they are. In other words, our ability to sit or stand still, to hold something without trembling or place ourselves in a position are assets of an organized and integrated neuromuscular (or we might say 'neuromyofascial') system.

INHIBITION

Two main types of inhibition occur in the nervous system – one is called 'presynaptic inhibition', and the other is 'postsynaptic inhibition'.

Presynaptic inhibition involves the activity of a presynaptic neuron (the neuron sending signals) being suppressed before it releases neurotransmitters at the synapse (the junction between two neurons). Gamma-aminobutyric acid (GABA) is the primary inhibitory neurotransmitter involved in presynaptic inhibition. When GABA is released by inhibitory interneurons onto the terminals of the presynaptic neuron, it binds to GABA receptors, leading to the following effects.

- Reduction in calcium influx. GABA binding reduces the influx of calcium ions into the presynaptic neuron. Calcium influx is necessary for the release of neurotransmitters. Therefore, reduced calcium entry results in fewer neurotransmitter vesicles being released into the synapse.
- Decreased neurotransmitter release. With fewer neurotransmitters released, there is a reduced likelihood of excitatory neurotransmitters (such as acetylcholine) binding to receptors on the postsynaptic neuron. This leads to decreased excitation of the postsynaptic neuron and, subsequently, muscle fibres.

Postsynaptic inhibition involves the inhibition of the postsynaptic neuron (the neuron receiving signals) by making it less responsive to excitatory signals. Glycine is the primary inhibitory neurotransmitter involved in postsynaptic inhibition, particularly in the spinal cord and brainstem. Glycine receptors are located on the postsynaptic neuron's membrane, and when glycine binds to these receptors, several effects occur.

- Increase in chloride influx. Glycine binding opens chloride channels on the postsynaptic neuron. Chloride ions flow into the neuron, hyperpolarizing it (making it more negative) and making it less likely to reach the threshold for firing an action potential.
- Reduced excitation. As the postsynaptic neuron becomes less excitable due to hyperpolarization, it becomes more resistant to excitatory signals from other neurons. This inhibition helps prevent excessive activation of muscle fibres and contributes to overall muscle control.

In both presynaptic and postsynaptic inhibition, the balance between excitatory and inhibitory neurotransmitters plays a crucial role in regulating *all* muscle activity – or all motion. This is a short segue to recognizing the importance of biomotional integrity, to use Avison's term (see Part 1). If the nervous system is synchronized appropriately, motion will be, too (regardless of modality).

The precise coordination of these inhibitory mechanisms ensures that muscles contract and are inhibited in a controlled manner, preventing spasms, tremors, and other unwanted or unnecessary movements. It is what makes a dancer's movements precise and what allows anyone to return a glass they have sipped from to the table, pick a blackberry, wipe their child's face or kiss them on the cheek to say goodnight, or place a key in a lock. That is what everyday movements rely on, for the smallest and slightest gestures. It is not only in peak performance or movement classes, that these integrating neuromyofascial expressions are exhibited. A smile, a wink, a wave to someone you love all incorporate these somewhat specialized, but nevertheless ordinary, coordinations and connections.

We often consider myofascial release to be something that becomes relevant in movement classes or performances. With that aspect in mind, I will mention safe range of motion and exactly what that is.

There are two specific kinds of range of motion (ROM) in the body:

1. physiological range of motion and
2. anatomical range of motion.

These terms refer to two different aspects of so-called joint movement in the human body, both of which are essential for understanding the capabilities and limitations of the myofascial system. They augment our full understanding of the term 'release' as applied to human motion.

Anatomical range of motion (ARM) refers to the *maximum extent to which a joint can move in its natural, anatomical structure* without being restricted by factors such as muscles, ligaments, tendons, and other surrounding tissues. Anatomical range of motion represents the *theoretical* limit of joint movement, considering only the joint's structural components. Anatomical range of motion is determined by the *shape* of the bones forming the joint, the *relationship* of those bones and the ligaments that stabilize the associated joint(s). It is a fixed measurement and doesn't account for the body's neuromuscular control or protective mechanisms that limit movement to prevent injury.

Physiological range of motion (PRM), on the other hand, refers to the range of movement that *a person can achieve* through voluntary muscle contractions and joint actions. This range is influenced by various factors beyond anatomical constraints, such as the neuromuscular efficiency and pliability of muscles, tendons, ligaments, as well as that person's nervous system's ability to control and coordinate movements. In other words, physiological range of motion accounts for the interaction between the musculo-skeletal and nervous systems (if we use these classical terms). The result of this brings us to the goal of biomotional intelligence: knowing the individual optimal range and sensing the self-organizing, natural capacity for movement that serves optimally. It is easy to under- or over-estimate (force and restrict) optimal individual physiological range of motion. This is where stretching can induce more PRM than a body can accommodate in the long-term. Young bodies over-stretching, as one example, can lead in later life to insufficient suitable stiffness to control precise movements. In other words, it can over force the stronger tissues in the body to become too lax for efficient movement or stillness in later life. It can impinge on the body's ability to relax comfortably when they are older, which is, effectively, taking the body beyond physiological range of motion.

There is a way to visualize this PRM quite clearly using a practical model as a helpful visual metaphor. Think of a Slinky®, a helical spring (see Figure 38). Hold a Slinky® in your hands. Take each end and press them together. Now, hold one end still while gently pulling with the other hand in the opposite direction, taking the ends of the Slinky® apart.

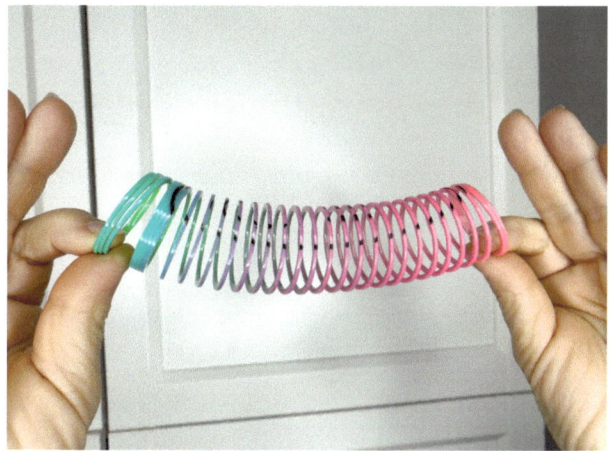

Figure 38

The Slinky® will elongate. If you release your pull on the Slinky® it will recoil and reform, or restore its original structure. That release and restore was free energy storage capacity; in other words, the structural elastic recoil of the spring-loaded design of a helical tube. All connective tissues, including fascia, myofascia etc. are organized in helical tubular patterns on every scale, from micro to macro.

Slinky®'s are even a great model for describing protein collagens in the human body, at the microscopic level. In this example, as the Slinky® elongates, one can really imagine a collagen protein elongating. Be careful not to elongate too far or you will permanently damage or disfigure the Slinky®.

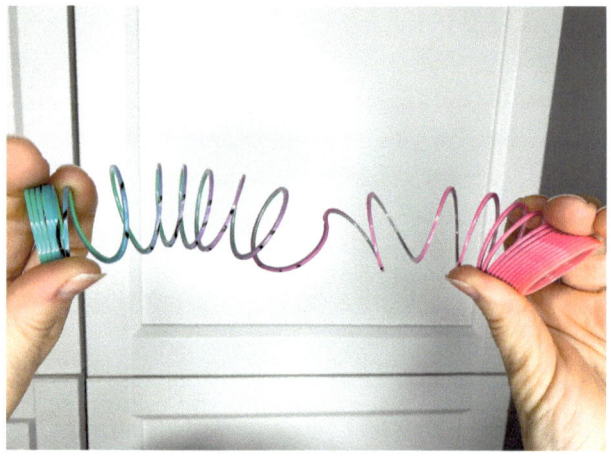

Figure 39

If you elongate the Slinky® too far (i.e., pulling it *beyond* its ability to spring back to its original position and shape) it will display something called plastic deformation and will never reform to its original shape and it will lose its integrity. In other words, it won't be able to release and restore *freely* as it did before. Its structural elastic recoil capacity will have been compromised (see Figure 39). This visually represents how tissues can be forced beyond PRM and permanently affected by the *imposed inability* to spring back.

For the purpose of our conversation, which is focusing on the word release, gather four or five of the spiral coils of the Slinky® between a finger and thumb and now compress them together (you may need a friend to help with this unless you have a third hand). Now when you pull on one end of the Slinky® you will notice the force ends at your fingers and the Slinky® beyond your fingers does not move or elongate. As an analogy for living connective tissues, pinching the four coils together is like having a scar or an adhesion in the tissue dampening the sharing of forces from one location to another, through the naturally free recoil system of the tissues. The forces are effectively blocked, or dampened.

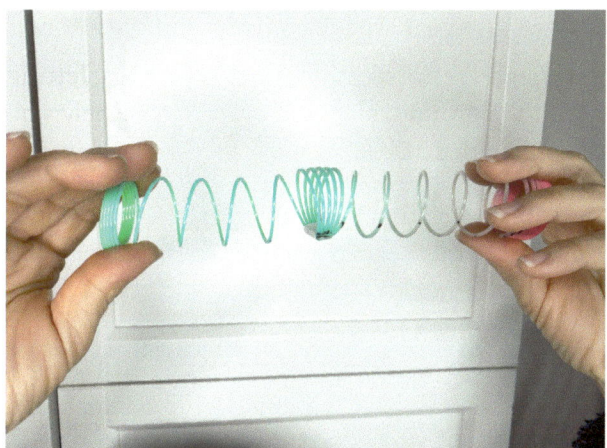

Figure 40

This model of a Slinky® correlates precisely, in dissection, with the tissues. For example, scarring can demonstrate readily how the surrounding tissues are compromised and 'dampened' in their physiological range of motion. The easiest way to imagine this is to imagine wearing a full body unitard that covered the head, too (think of a Spider-Man suit). If there was a split anywhere in the suit that was then stitched up over an area to bind it together (like a scar), the 'pull' would be felt (to one extent or another) throughout the body. It may be particularly keen at the major joints – particularly neighbouring ones – where any dampening or restriction would affect their natural range by 'pulling' on the fold at such a place elsewhere in the body (see Figure 40).

What we call 'release' in the human body, then, has something to do with preserving our physiological range of motion with the integrity that matches our own body. That might include ensuring that any joint in the body is honoured. Forcing length or ignoring compression can both come at a cost. If that is considered in terms of the Slinky®, it would be like 'leaving it stuck' in its immobile 'closed' state, or pulling on it too much, so that it cannot restore its closed state, in process of responding by (albeit apparently) lengthening again. What we are referring to is an appropriate range of motion that activates and inhibits naturally, within our tissue matrix.

When we are walking, we look to one leg to be relatively active and the other to be appropriately 'inhibited' as they switch and coordinate according to the rhythm and requirements of that movement; restoring as they move. In Wilbour Kelsick's contribution on rebound, we learn how differently these coordinating sequences express themselves in more complex movements such as hurdling. In both walking, hurdling, or any such motions, the coordination we seek relies on all the Rs and particularly rhythm for the useful resonance they can confer on the human body system. The innate recoil and the effective refinement of the tissues to promote these deep essential resources of human motion are all contributing factors to well-being.

My view of the human body could be described as a Monism view, that is, your body and my body represent a seamless whole. Deep to your skin exists an inner cosmos that is unified from before birth to beyond death. That said, it could, therefore, be possible to work in one region of the body and experience a feeling of release in another because the body is not bureaucratic, atomistic, rigid, or disembodied or disconnected, anywhere. It is continuous, connected; it is one.

Restore

Helen Eadie

TO RESTORE

To 'restore' is to facilitate the return of an intrinsic condition, quality, or ability. It implies the reestablishment of wholeness, a giving back of something. It's an act of care, love, empathy, compassion and above all attentiveness, whether it's the Sistine Chapel, a sense of hope, or your health that requires restoration.

> *Experience is never limited, and it is never complete; it is an immense sensibility, a kind of huge spider-web of the finest silken threads suspended in the chamber of consciousness, and catching every air-borne particle in its tissue.*
>
> (Henry James)[12]

So, what exactly are we restoring when it comes to myofascia? If we take this question at face value our immediate response might be 'health', 'tensional integrity', 'elasticity', and/or 'optimal performance'. All of which is true, but is there more to myofascia than its material properties?

> *What I see in Nature is a magnificent structure that we can comprehend only very imperfectly, and that must fill a thinking person with a feeling of humility.*
>
> (Albert Einstein)[13]

---

12   James, H. (1884) 'The Art of Fiction.' London: *Longman's Magazine*.
13   Stefan, V. A. (2002) *Einstein's Revolutionary Wisdom.* San Diego, CA: Stefan University Press.

To fully appreciate the depths of this question we must step outside the box of Western scientific dogma, and lightly examine the assumptions and unconscious biases of a system which positions itself as the harbinger of truth.

As Joanne has already established, the study of human anatomy has remained within a materialist paradigm for the last 400 years. The biomedical model (the most pervasive and influential model of physical health in Western culture) views the body as a biological material organism, which can be understood through the reductive process of examining its constituent parts.

This 'way of seeing' feeds into the wider materialist philosophy; that the universe is built up from discrete component parts into more complex structures; and that it exists independently of and is ontologically prior (existing at a more fundamental level) to mind/consciousness.

That last sentence is *huge*! There is a built-in assumption to biological science which proposes reality as fundamentally material, and consciousness as secondary, a sort of by-product of the material brain. This theory is so insidious within Western culture, it reminds me of David Foster Wallace's fish parable:

> *There are these two young fish swimming along, and they happen to meet an older fish swimming the other way, who nods at them and says, 'Morning, boys. How's the water?' And the two young fish swim on for a bit, and then eventually one of them looks over at the other and goes, 'What the hell is water?'*[14]

In the West, we swim within materialist waters. It's a prevailing narrative so entrenched in our everyday ideas and thinking that we've lost sight of the fact that it's a hypothesis. It's not the absolute truth. According to neuroscientist and psychiatrist Iain McGilchrist, seeing the world in terms of discrete inanimate, component parts, is a symptom of how the left hemisphere of our brain conceives reality. The wider implication of this statement suggests that the structure of our awareness creates the structure of our world – but more on that later.[15]

---

14   Wallace, D. F. (2009) *This is Water: Some Thoughts, Delivered on a Significant Occasion, about Living a Compassionate Life.* New York: Little, Brown and Company.
15   McGilchrist, I. (2019) *The Master and His Emissary: The Divided Brain and the Making of the Western World.* 2nd edition. New Haven, CT: Yale University Press.

Within the materialist paradigm, myofascia is categorized as a material 'thing', that in essence is void of consciousness/mind. According to this worldview, what we'd be restoring to our myofascia would necessarily be its material properties (e.g., elasticity) and, therefore, be causally dependent on a physical process.

Can you see how the underlying structure of Western science funnels our method of questioning down a particular material rabbit hole, and thus reinforces such ideas through the responding 'results' of that scientific enquiry?

Just to be clear, I'm not saying if you're interested in the material properties of fascia, you therefore subscribe to the dogma of reductionist materialism. Just that we ought to be aware of its credulity and limitations, as both a philosophy and scientific method when we ask questions about our living architecture.

The physical health of our myofascia is extremely important, and appropriate training and rest is instrumental in helping us restore tissue integrity and optimal performance. As an area of research and interest, it rightly deserves the scrutiny science has bestowed upon it. The point I'm trying to make here is that this perspective of restore – one that focuses on the material aspects of myofascia – is just one part of a much bigger picture.

WHAT CAN OTHER FRAMEWORKS SHOW US?

So, what are we restoring to myofascia if it's not material? Are there other frameworks we can address this question in, and how might that yield a different response? What if we ask the question within a paradigm that values consciousness – not matter – as the fundamental essence of existence?

Many scientists, especially those working in the field of quantum physics, conclude that consciousness is primary to matter. Sir James Jeans, a physicist, astronomer, and mathematician stated in the early twentieth century that:

Knowledge is heading towards a non-mechanical reality; the universe begins to look more like a great thought than like a great machine. Mind no longer appears to be an accidental intruder into the realm of matter...we ought rather to hail it as the creator and governor of the realm of matter.[16]

Another powerful statement from theoretical physicist and Nobel Prize winner, Max Planck, should have us stop in our tracks and wonder:

As a physicist, and therefore as a man who has spent his whole life in service of the most down-to-earth science, namely the exploration of matter, no one is going to take me for a starry-eyed dreamer. After all my exploration of the atom, then, let me tell you this; there is no matter as such. All matter arises and exists only by virtue of a force which sets the atomic particles oscillating...we must suppose, behind this force, a conscious, intelligent spirit. This spirit is the ultimate origin of matter.[17]

Scientist and complexity theorist Neil Theise, who introduced the concept of the interstitium (the continuous web of space that exists between fascia fibres) to the fascia community at the 2018 International Fascia Research Congress, proposes in his paper 'Fundamental Awareness', co-written with colleague Menas Kafatos, that fundamental awareness (awareness of awareness) is the essence of all reality. Regarding the everyday physical world we experience, they write: '"thingness", the appearance of materiality, even of living things, is dependent on the scale of observation.'[18]

Theise draws on complexity theory to reveal that 'things' are not the solid fixed entities we assume them to be, but are in fact different scales of self-organizing phenomena:

In self-organizing systems, whether the entities involved appear to be a thing versus a process arising from the interaction of smaller things depends on the level of scale at which the system is observed. Thus, a bait ball of fish appears as an object, a 'ball', at this level of scale, though it is clear from closer observation that the ball is made of interacting fish; likewise, the fish themselves appear as solid entities

16   Jeans, Sir J. (1931) *The Mysterious Universe*. 2nd edition. Cambridge: Cambridge University Press.

17   Planck, M. (1959) *The New Science: 3 Complete Works: Where is Science Going? The Universe in the Light of Modern Physics; The Philosophy of Physics*. New York: Meridian Books.

18   Theise, N. D. and Kafatos, M. C. (2016) 'Fundamental awareness: A framework for integrating science, philosophy and metaphysics.' *Communicative and Integrative Biology* 9, 3, e1155010.

at the everyday scale, but are recognized as emergent phenomena of interacting cells at the microscope level.[19]

The words 'self-organizing' and 'emergent' are terms Joanne uses to describe the becoming of the embryo, as it forms itself through the weaving of its own fascial web. Planck's 'spirit', Theise and Kafatos's 'fundamental awareness', or we could just say consciousness, is generating and governing the growth and formation of the embryo at multiple scales. From an energetic field, into a liquid base, it emerges as a myofascia form, with all our cognitive capacities, and a deep impulse to love, be loved, and connect. According to this paradigm, we emerge out of consciousness.

Let us assume that consciousness is primary, organizing and sustaining our matter; what then is the relationship between our myofascia and metaphysical selves, i.e., our experience as conscious beings? Can the relationship between consciousness and myofascia be compromised? And if so, how can it be restored?

OUR INTEROCEPTIVE WORLD

How do we know we're conscious? What gives us the sense that we are alive and aware? Let's first distinguish fundamental consciousness from individual consciousness. They're not separate but neither are they the same. We can think of our own individual consciousness as an expression or manifestation of a fundamental consciousness.

This idea can be presented metaphorically through the body. The trillions of cells that make up our material body are essentially derived from one cell (us as a unicellular organism). They're generated from the body, are of the body, replicate functions of the body (respiration, metabolization, etc.) and yet each cell is its own body, distinct with individual purpose.

McGilchrist proposes a beautiful idea, that matter is itself a phase of consciousness, not a temporal phase, but a textural phase along a continuum, like the seamless solid–gel–liquid–vapour phases of water.[20] According to him, matter acts as a creative force of *resistance*, through

---

19   Ibid.
20   McGilchrist, I. (2021) *The Matter with Things: Our Brains, Our Delusions, and the Unmaking of the World*. UK: Perspectiva Press.

which the fundamental force of conscious potential expresses itself as perceived through the biological kingdoms of our planet and the mysterious structures of space.

Our pre-tensioned architecture is itself inherently resistant, self-strung, as it were, into a multidimensional web. Unlike the dwelling of a spider, however, our myofascial net and the spaces within the net, are innervated with sensory nerves that continuously stream information in the form of chemicals and, for want of a better word, 'mechanical' tension to our brain. Some of this sensory information we're consciously aware of, some of it we're not. The term that has been coined to describe this phenomenon is 'interoception'.

Robert Schleip distinguishes interoception from proprioception.

The term interoception is usually applied to describe body perceptions that are less concerned with where our body is in space and in relation to gravity, and more with how it is doing in its constant search for homeostasis related to our physiological needs. Interoception signalling is therefore associated with somatic perceptions, such as temperature changes, hunger, thirst, nausea, tingling, soreness, oxygen supply, and muscular effort, as well as a sense of belonging (versus alienation) regarding specific body regions.[21]

He then goes on to explain that:

The peripheral sensory receptors related to interoception are all free nerve endings – they are interstitial receptors. Most of those receptors are located in visceral connective tissues.[22]

Drawing on the collective work of Schleip, Findley, Chaitow, and Huijing, Bordoni and Marelli state that: '*the receptors that send information about interoception are not only located in the viscera but also in the myofascial areas of the trunk and limbs.*'[23] Our myofascial bodies are the very substrate of our 'felt sense'.

21   Schleip, R. (2022) 'The fascial network.' *Massage and Bodywork Magazine for the Visually Impaired 37*, 5.
22   Ibid.
23   Bordoni, B. and Marelli, F. (2017) 'Emotions in motion: myofascial interoception.' *Complementary Medicine Research 24*, 110–113.

Tsakiris and Critchley, both respective professors within the fields of psychiatry and psychology state that *'interoceptive processes can enhance the accounts of mechanisms that underpin affective* [attitudes and emotions elicited by a stimulus] *and cognitive functions, including the coherent representation of a conscious sense of self.'*[24]

In other words, feelings from our 'inner sense' motivate our behaviours and emotions to maintain physiological integrity. Most of these processes happen at an unconscious level, but we do have the capacity to consciously train our interoceptive awareness. Why is that? And what are the effects of doing so?

HEART

It has been demonstrated that people with good metacognitive awareness (awareness of one's own thought processes) of their heartbeat (one quantitative measure of interoception) are better protected against experiencing anxiety.[25]

No wonder cardioception, i.e., the felt sense of our heartbeat, is a primary source and measure of interoceptive awareness. The heart is incredibly fundamental to our body formation, organization, general health, and sense of self. At the earliest stages of our development, its relentless beat danced us into existence. Dr Michael Shea, a psychologist and biodynamic craniosacral therapist writes in his book *The Heart of the Practice*:

> *The heart is the single most common centre of the human body for all growth and development primarily because it is the primary source of nutrition for internal growth once it becomes operational around three weeks post fertilization...the heart and its own autonomous nervous and endocrine systems co-regulate deeper structures of the brain.*[26]

24 Tsakiris, M. and Critchley, H. (2016) 'Interoception beyond homeostasis: affect, cognition and mental health.' *Philosophical Transactions of the Royal Society of London, Series B, Biological sciences 371*, 1708, 20160002.
25 Ibid.
26 Shea, M. J. (2016) *Biodynamic Craniosacral Therapy: The Heart of the Practice*. CreateSpace Independent Publishing Platform.

The HeartMath Institute conducts leading edge research on the physio-logical and emotional intelligence of the heart. They've developed tools and techniques, rooted in evidence-based research that help people tap into their heart intelligence, to improve self-regulation, overall health, cognitive function, and performance.[27]

The method involves cardioception, breath awareness, attention, and sustained positive emotions (particularly gratitude), to intentionally influence the heart's rhythmic patterns and heart rate variability (HRV). Those who practise the Buddhist meditation Metta, otherwise known as loving-kindness meditation, will be familiar with the HeartMath practice known as heart-centred breathing.

The practice of heart-centred breathing has a systemic effect on the whole person, leading to objective and measurable improvements in physiological and behavioural functioning, along with subjective feelings of coherence, calm, and deep connection.[28]

Awareness is at the heart of the practice (pun intended), and so it would seem that conscious connection to your heart yields many health and well-being benefits. It serves us to remember that the heart is part of – albeit highly specialized – our myofascia matrix, formed under tension and held within our wider web. Restoring myofascia magic is as much about heart connection as it is anything else.

Other contemplative practices (such as yoga and craniosacral ther-apy), which invite you to slow down, to notice, to observe, and to listen, are also opening up the possibility for you to tune into and attune your interoceptive system.

Dr Helen Weng at the University of California San Francisco says:

Researchers and clinicians are recognizing interoception as a key mechanism to mental and physical health, where understanding our body's signals helps us understand and regulate emotional and physical states.[29]

In contrast to good metacognitive awareness of our internal sensory world, interoceptive dysregulation has been associated with eating

27 Heartmath.org
28 Ibid.
29 Robson, D. (2021) 'Interoception: the hidden sense that shapes wellbeing.' *The Observer Science,* 15 August, 2021.

disorders, post-traumatic stress disorder (PTSD), depression, anxiety, autism spectrum disorders, fibromyalgia, and chronic fatigue syndrome.[30]

As you can see, interoception is foundational to our physical, emotional, and psychological health. It seems that listening to our body (via the myofascia matrix, embellished as it is with hundreds of millions of free nerve endings communicating sensory information to our brain)[31] helps us take better care of our mind.

Physical practices which foster interoceptive awareness require attention and the ability to slow down, to be with what is. Alongside the already-mentioned yoga, meditation, and craniosacral therapy, other practices include tai chi, Feldenkrais, somatic movement, body–mind centring, continuum, and undoubtedly many more.

There is an important distinction to make between interoception and proprioception when considering the types of movement practices we might engage with to restore myofascial magic. As Robert Schleip has noted:

> *The neural stimulation from those interoceptive nerve endings does not follow the usual afferent [information carried towards the central nervous system] pathways toward the somatomotor cortex in the brain; rather these neurons project to the so-called insular cortex.[32]*

Essentially, signals from our interoceptive and proprioceptive system communicate to the central nervous system through different pathways and are organized differently in the brain. Why does this matter? Well, if we tend to bias movement or exercise that leans into the high-intensity, high-speed, high-performance end of the spectrum, or is heavily focused on form in space, without a mindful component that invites listening, we fail to nourish the highest proportion of our sensory receptors, those that constitute our interoceptive world. The key message being different sensory nerves require different forms of stimulation.

We have far more interoceptive nerves than we do proprioceptive nerves, meaning our capacity to feel within is far greater than our capacity to sense where we are in space. The majority of our interoceptive nerves are low threshold receptors which are '*responsive to mechanical*

30 Schleip, 'The fascial network.'
31 Ibid.
32 Ibid.

tension, pressure, or shear deformation.[33] They are exquisitely sensitive, responsive to the lightest touch and most subtle of movements.

This is where a physical practice not only gets really interesting, but deeply therapeutic, transcending the realms of fitness and performance, into the subtle, qualitative internal world of micro-movement. It's where we shift our attention from 'how do I look' to 'how do I feel'.

Our myofascial–interstitial–interoceptive–galaxy of free nerve endings, communicates with a specific part of our brain – the insular cortex – which evidence suggests is the gateway to self-conscious awareness.[34] If consciousness precedes matter, and is the fundamental essence of all reality, could stimulating our insular cortex through interoceptive practices not only *enrich* our sense of phenomenal consciousness but also be the gateway into fundamental consciousness from which everything derives? How might that energy source feel? Does it have distinct qualities?

Are the undeniable feelings of centredness, calm, connectedness, coherence, and pure presence that we experience after engaging in interoceptive practices, simply us tapping into and channelling a greater source of awareness that exists beyond and predicates our subjective selves?

BRAIN

Earlier I mentioned neuroscientist, psychiatrist, and all-round polymath Iain McGilchrist. The breadth and depth of his work goes way beyond the scope of my contribution here, but what I can share is, I think, significant and relevant to the conversation around interoception, consciousness, and the fascia matrix.

He stands with other scientists in positing that consciousness is the fundamental source of reality. His fascinating hypothesis, built on decades of neuroscience research and clinical experience, proposes that the left hemisphere and the right hemisphere of the human brain attend

33   Schleip, R. and Jäger, H. (2012) 'Interoception. A new correlate for intricate connections between fascial receptors, emotion and self-recognition.' In Schleip, R., Findley, T. W., Chaitow, L. and Huijing, P. A. (eds) *Fascia: The Tensional Network of the Human Body*. Edinburgh: Churchill Livingstone/Elsevier.
34   Huang, Z., Tarnal, V., Vlisides, P. E., Janke, E. L. *et al.* (2021) 'Anterior insula regulates brain network transitions that gate conscious access.' *Cell Reports 35*, 5, 109081.

to the world in completely separate ways. This is not to be confused with the popular yet inaccurate myth that the left and right brain have completely distinct functions, i.e., left deals with reason, right with creativity – the truth is that both hemispheres participate in all brain functions. What McGilchrist encourages us towards is how they differ, as opposed to what the difference is; it's a subtle yet powerful distinction.

McGilchrist states that each hemisphere perceives reality differently, as a direct result of the way each attends to the world. Sound familiar? Let's use the materialist argument as an example. If you assert that matter is fundamental and devoid of consciousness, then it follows through that the questions you ask regarding the what, how, and whys of the world will align with your ideology. There is no talk of 'spirit' or 'fundamental consciousness' in classical anatomy.

The different structures of awareness in both hemispheres determine what it is we 'see' as our reality. And although both hemispheres bring value to our experience, and indeed must work together for optimal performance, McGilchrist asserts that 'as far as attention and perception go, the right hemisphere is a more important guide and more reliable one to the nature of reality.'[35]

It turns out that it is the right hemisphere which is more in touch with the body and is better able to regulate our emotions. Thinking back to how interoceptive nerves communicate with the insular cortex (the gateway to consciousness), it's interesting to note that it's specifically *right* insula mediated. And that it is the right hemisphere that predominates in receiving and interpreting information from the heart.[36]

McGilchrist writes:

> The experimental self, the self in the present moment, the self-sensing what is occurring on one's thoughts, feelings and body state, without purpose or goal, other than noticing how things are from one moment to the next, the self that is recruited by mindfulness, is associated with widespread right hemisphere activations.[37]

Regions of the right hemisphere process our perception of biological

35   McGilchrist, *The Matter with Things: Our Brains, Our Delusions, and the Unmaking of the World.*
36   Ibid.
37   Ibid.

motion and whole-body motion. And how we move in the world, in turn, affects our perception. If our posture is slumped and we walk tentatively with our eyes to the ground, this will inevitably affect our perception of self, and the environment around us. Likewise, if we perceive the world as a scary, hostile, and meaningless place, this will undoubtedly affect how we move through it.

Below is a diagram to illustrate the differences of how each hemisphere attends to the world, based on the descriptions used by McGilchrist. The blue hemisphere represents the right brain, the red hemisphere the left brain, depicting the opposite characteristics of each.

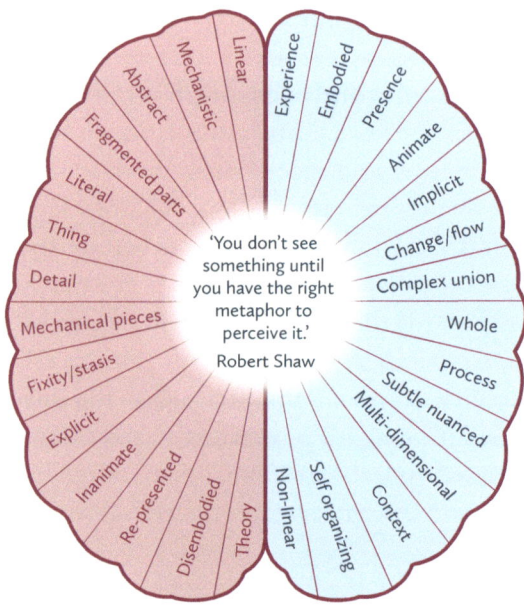

Figure 41 Left and right brain chart.
Adapted from the work of Iain McGilchrist by Helen Eadie, image by Bex Hawkins. Reproduced with permission from Helen Eadie.

If, like McGilchrist asserts, the right hemisphere is a closer, more reliable guide to the nature of reality, does this mean training our interoceptive awareness (which is processed by the right hemisphere) helps us become more conscious of reality as it really is, in all its flowing, interconnected wholeness? Does *how* we practice shape *how* we see the world?

Inversely, can a worldview that biases the attentional qualities of one hemisphere affect how we move and relate to our body? For example, if my worldview preferences the attentional style of the left hemisphere, how might this affect how I move, perceive, and feel my body?

The quote from Robert Stetson Shaw in the centre of the illustration nicely sums up how McGilchrist's hemisphere hypothesis serves as a metaphor for classical (left hemisphere) and contemporary (right hemisphere) models of human anatomy and movement. Classical anatomy germinated in the industrial revolution, but was this underpinned by a Western cultural bias towards left hemisphere attention?

Is our recognition of the fascia matrix as a sensory, multidimensional whole, a sign that we are collectively shifting towards a right hemisphere worldview, aligning our understanding of the human body with the nature of reality?

NOVELTY

As we have seen, the type of attention we deploy matters. It literally changes our phenomenal experience. Seemingly then, right hemisphere attention is of great value to how we practice movement. McGilchrist again:

> wide-open, vigilant, sustained attention of right hemisphere, without preconception as to what it may find...more exploratory, less certain: it is more interested in making discriminations, in shades of meaning. Its attention, one might say, is not so much linear as in the round.[38]

Yes, you read that correctly, the suggestion that right hemisphere attention is round; just as Joanne's proclamation that the breath is round, and the body is round. How neat! This kind of attention fosters novelty, giving us the opportunity to be truly present to sensations as they unfold. This is such a valuable practice because it disrupts habitual patterns.

Neuroscientist Dr Lisa Feldman Barrett says that our brain predicts (almost) everything we do: 'Your brain is wired to initiate your actions *before* you're aware of them...your brain predicts and prepares your actions using your past experiences.'[39]

---

38   Ibid.
39   Barrett, L. F. (2021) *Seven and a Half Lessons About the Brain*. Boston, MA: Mariner Books.

This predictive phenomenon is happening all the time, and for the most part we're totally unaware of it. The downside to what is otherwise an incredible superpower is that the brain's predictions are not always right. When it comes to movement and body perception, we might unconsciously hold ourselves in inertial patterns with predictions (which the brain has coded from accumulated habits and prior experiences, no longer relevant to who we are today, right now in this moment) running the show.

Although we can't change our past to affect our predictions, we can disrupt the process. The technical term for a mismatch between prior expectations and reality within the brain is called 'prediction error'. These 'blips' create an opportunity to change and fine tune our brain's predictions. All this neural tweaking happens 'under the hood', without us being aware of it.

So how do we consciously probe the brain's predictive nature, to connect with the raw sensations of our body, in pursuit of expanding our phenomenal experience, and disrupting old and redundant habits? The answer lies in novelty, the precursor of which, according to McGilchrist, is that 'wide-open, vigilant, sustained attention of right hemisphere, without preconception as to what it may find'.[40]

In this attentional space we get to *experience* the distinction and know the difference that is *thinking* about our body (based on memories, predictions, images) and *feeling* the raw sensations of our bodies, as they arise from our body, via fascial pathways, in communion with our brain.

Attending to ourselves in this receptive, no expectations, broad awareness manner, helps to consciously feed present moment sensations to our brain, giving it the opportunity to refine and change predictions that have run their due course. It's not always easy; it takes practice, patience, and tolerance to 'not know'. Yet with time we get more skilled at listening, our sensory experiences become further granulated, which in turn trains our capacity for discernment and refinement, skills we can apply not only to our movement practices but to everyday life.

---

40 McGilchrist, *The Matter with Things: Our Brains, Our Delusions, and the Unmaking of the World.*

SLOW IT DOWN

Slowing down is an essential component for cultivating open, vigilant, sustained attention. The relationship between speed and attention is a curious one. It's true that we can be in a flow state *whilst* doing something at speed; think Olympic 100 m champions. Yet slowing down movement *also* alchemizes our attention, altering our consciousness of time to the point where we are completely absorbed in the flow of our moment-to-moment sensations. Slowing down helps us capture novelty as it arises in conscious awareness.

And what's more, your body knows when it's being listened to. The more you practice tuning in to your sensory self, the more your bodily intelligence rises to the surface of your awareness. The feeling of being in sensory communion with the body, whether it's my own or a client's, often feels like communication with a gentle creature. It's an alive intelligence which precedes conditioning, ego, and personality. It's veridical and spirited, and it flows.

Slowed movement, awareness and use of ground, gravity, and guided force transmission, is food for your fascial free nerve endings, the majority of which respond to subtle, light touch, and motion. An interoceptive practice invites us to mindfully move and slowly tension the tissues, directing force distribution through the densities and pathways of our myofascial matrix, enlivening the tissue and our sense of self as we go.

Myofascia magic is remembering that we are always 'becoming', more so than we are simply 'being'. It's restoring the awareness that we are not fixed, mechanical, and made of parts, no matter how entrenched that myth is within Western culture. We are flowing, self-organizing, non-linear processes, with boundless hearts and minds.

Refine

Paul Thornley

Refining movement is a continuous conscious journey spanning the entire lifetime. It is a process; one that will have long-lasting effects across many and various aspects of everyday life. Movement can be like medicine if it is understood. It is not acting as medicine when rehabilitation and external medical *intervention* are required, due to detrimental movement patterns. Often this can arise simply through patterns that have been taken for granted, without knowledge of the consequences and ramifications those particular movement choices can have.

Many people naturally take the ability to move for granted, just as it is possible to take the ability to heal during our early years for granted. There is a licence in knowing these incredible human bodies can and do adapt every moment of every day; it is a gift nature gives many individuals. There is an acquired skill in understanding *how* the body adapts, and learning that there is unlimited positive influence over the *way* it adapts. Lesson one in that skill is recognizing that there is a threshold of 'negative adaptation'. Once identified, that ceiling that cannot be breached, it gives each individual a conscious constraint. It may not be entirely pleasant to discover at first, as the sensations that go with it include having to endure the discomfort and limitations that come as a cost of not being aware. However, once that moment of 'knowing you've taken it too far' comes, there is a huge value in recognizing and distinguishing that personal constraint. It serves as a powerful feedback loop to discovering and deepening the practices that work individually, and the personalized way in which they enhance adaptation ongoingly.

It could be considered as a kind of alchemy, whereby the 'lead of the wound' is transformed into the 'gold of the gift'. It's something more than 'knowing the limitations'. It is a powerful container of adaptability that, once stored in the library of tissue awareness, once it is refined, it becomes a deep and resilient resource.

The practice then gives back something much greater than the sum of the parts. By recognizing the importance of movement *quality* and embracing a practice of myofascial magic in action that will enhance it, individuals can unlock the potential for new qualities in the body that it can add to that library of resources day in and day out. They include balance, precision, resilience, control, and grace that ensure the longevity of choice that everyone desires. Losing that choice, that aspect of adaptability, becomes extremely expensive when it costs freedom of movement and, even inadvertently, builds in training repertoires that become repetitive strain injuries over time! Everyone has habitual patterns that don't necessarily serve them, so this focus allows new and beneficial habits to be gently introduced like a 'dose and degree movement medicine' that deepens the awareness, while it resources the archive of valuable patterns.

All the five Rs of myofascial magic in action are paramount in the management of our movement effects. They are designed, in practice, to take the body from larger, more general movements to more subtle integration. Refine, the subject of this section, is the cornerstone of the whole set. It brings forward a magical ingredient that establishes a body that will not require the preceding Rs as often. In some ways, it requires the most focus to establish; however, the rewards bring benefits that become a deep asset to moving well in life, every day. It doesn't offer a new sport, or a different movement modality. It feeds the connective tissue body with structural awareness that enhances the optimum adaptability and appropriateness of response. What is meant by that is that *when the unexpected happens,* the body simply responds, rapidly and appropriately at the time. Whatever the main movement modality (such as yoga, Pilates, martial art, dance, personal training, gym sessions, what-ever it is) the myofascial magic in action movements in Refine ensure that no unhelpful movement patterns are being inadvertently driven into the tissue organization. This can result in sudden inadvertent injuries that can easily be avoided when the movement medicine is right for the body that's moving.

It doesn't just apply to sports and fitness or named activities. Whether on the sports field, stage, or in the realm of everyday activities, the pur-suit of refined movement contributes to a more fulfilled and empowered existence. Movement is an integral part of our existence, and its refinement holds the key to enhanced functionality, performance, and overall well-being. It goes much deeper than quantifiable measures of physical achievement. It brings an inner confidence, a kind of self-knowing of inner balance, a deeper self-sense that seems to occur just through the subtle practices of this section.

In a world of extremes, it is vital to embrace subtlety. It may look easy; it may even seem less important than the more intensive exercise programmes that are usually adopted for sports and training sessions. However, this change of intensity is the answer to attaining and maintaining longevity of choice in all the other movements. It is the foundation of everything else. Honing the quality and precision of our movements can yield remarkable benefits. Incorporating myofascial magic in action has demonstrably increased the impact and difference of training in a variety of movement modalities. Evidently, through feedback from teachers in various styles of yoga, Pilates, martial arts, and other practices, understanding movement refinement is at the heart of creating a better and more fulfilling life for themselves and their clients. It really deepens the ability to control the movement outcomes they and their clients are likely to face in day-to-day living and management.

Movement refinement involves the process of optimizing and enhancing the quality of every move. It encompasses physical, mental, and emotional aspects that influence the way we execute actions, whether they are basic daily activities or specialized skills. This is not limited to movement teachers. Consider that dancers, actors, musicians, nurses, doctors and professionals of every stripe (not to exclude non-professional roles of parents and people of every age group) all depend on refined movement to convey emotions and narratives. Whether a medic is performing surgery, or an optician is testing eyes, or a lecturer is on stage performing an educational presentation, the body is moving. Every gesture, step, or note is carefully honed to achieve the desired impact on the audience or client, or patient. Practicing movement precision allows all kinds of performers to deliver captivating and authentic expressions. Every gesture resonates with the theme of refinement, and it enhances everything they do.

As instructors, trainers, and coaches, we have to be somewhat like the conductor of an orchestra, an orchestra that is comprised of many different instruments, all to one degree or another slightly out of tune.

Our role is to refine them all individually, address each of their unique characteristics that ensure they are finely tuned to perform at their optimal best. Then they have to work as a collective, so the refinement can be taken to the next level of resilience.

This is the art of refining movement. It requires many subtle aspects. For example, all the players, their unique instruments, the music (including volume, tone, tempo) are all aspects of the language that is used to promote refinement. It is critical to learn observation and listening, in the context of these relatively simple and powerful movements. They can endorse *the individual's* own ability to reap the benefits of refinement reliably and sustainably. It is worth the effort to express our observations in the same language they understand, honouring their movement patterns. We can explain our interpretations and descriptions of what we have noticed. We can suggest appropriately how we are going to make those delicious refinements to maximize the individual's ability to move effortlessly.

In athletics, refined movement is essential for peak performance and at elite levels it can often be focused on intensity. Athletes train tirelessly to fine-tune their techniques and optimize their spring-loaded stored energy capacity. (We refer to that as optimizing fasciategrity; see Part 3). They also seek to cultivate myofascial memory and ensure highly potent movement patterns. From a basketball player's perfect jump shot to a gymnast's graceful routine, refining movement in sports often leads to greater consistency and reduced risk of injury.

Refinement, like everything, is specific to the time frame and the choices offered by each environment. They can often dictate the outcome. As such, elite sports performers often have short careers. They can become so finely tuned, that their bodies reach that ceiling of negative adaptation much earlier than someone from the public enjoying the same activity at considerably lower intensity. For all abilities there is a unique requirement to be able to perform and compete at the appropriate level. The type of refinement will reflect that specificity. It is a question often asked, as the understanding of the fascia matrix and its profound relationship to time and timing becomes more understood, if less intensity and higher refinement (they are not synonymous) might change the longevity of elite sportsmanship. It isn't rare to see young, promising athletes stopped in their intended careers while still in their teens, by injury and disenchantment. Is it worth considering that restoring, recovering, and resting play as powerful a role as refinement in the pursuit of long-term adaptability and consistent high-level performance?

For most of us, it is in everyday activities that we can benefit most from refined movement. Great posture serves everyday life movements such as carrying shopping, walking a dog, getting in and out of a car, sitting at a desk, lifting something down from or up to a shelf, picking something up off the floor, and so on. Efficient myofascial organization and fasciategrity in motion will contribute to improved energy conservation and reduced strain on the body. It really is like building an archive of reserve in terms of range, mobility, and adaptability. The approach of movement refinement can enhance overall well-being and prevent chronic issues stemming from poor movement quality in the first place.

Awareness of the body's sensory nature, the foundation of the latest research in fascia science, is essential for recognizing inner proprioception (interoception). In a world of distraction, having clarity and confidence removes confusion and clumsiness. These deliberate, conscious practices involve breaking down movements into smaller micro-movements, addressing what are called 'inhibiting effects' with their accompanying bias and gradually integrating improved structural integrity.

There are multiple positive benefits of practicing refined movement protocols to enhance the body's natural robustness (rather than ignoring it and finding out through unexpected injury that the crucial limit has been reached). It reduces the likelihood of injuries by minimizing unnecessary strain on the body and setting up a positive feedback loop promoting the body's innate adaptation abilities. The more appropriate techniques distribute forces more efficiently and performance becomes noticeably easier and, by default, more efficient. In some ways it is like revealing a secret 'less is more' code to release an innate ability that many people don't realize they have. It isn't 'any less is any more'; it is very specific and, as said previously, the crucial part is learning (as a movement teacher) how to identify the optimum dialect for the body language of a particular client. It is a learnable skill, and it is such a valuable one. With practice it becomes progressively easier to distinguish exactly 'what and how much less' is required and precisely 'what more' can be relinquished. The results are usually surprising and super valuable. As the conductor, it becomes possible to tune a whole orchestra in a relatively large classroom and inspire more refined movements for larger groups of individuals as well as one-to-one clients.

Refined movement is efficient movement, whether you are an athlete aiming for a personal best or an office worker striving for productivity, well-honed movement patterns lead to increased efficiency and optimal performance in all walks of life. When such naturally refined movement becomes second nature, individuals exude confidence and presence. This is evident in the grace and poise displayed by performers and athletes who have truly mastered their craft.

THE GOLDEN RULE OF REFINEMENT

Form governs Function and Function governs Form.

People do not really have 'bad posture'. Rather they have inefficient movement patterns, or they knowingly choose suboptimal movement choices and then deal with the effects of them. They also may have injuries and insults that force certain adaptations. It is often a moveable feast to some extent, if you know that the shape you have become determines the effectiveness and ease of any movement you attempt. It can be a self-fulfilling prophecy (excluding certain conditions, serious injury, and disability) rather than a default condition that nothing can be done about. In a healthy, mobile body, the way someone moves will dictate the way the body adapts and creates the shape that person lives with.

Making great movement choices, getting informed, understanding what you are asking of yourself, and knowing how you are going about achieving that motion are all crucial elements of being able to hone and adapt and improve (essentially refine) the body and the movement.

This is a combination of understanding twenty-first century anatomy, structure, and functionality. Integrating this knowledge into tried and tested (and frankly phenomenal movement options) brings myofascial magic to every action. It enhances the longevity we all seek from our incredible bodies in a world that daily challenges our ability to survive, let alone thrive.

Understanding what you are made of from an embryonic development and how you have created and grown yourself into the incredible being you are today, will allow you to focus more appropriately when endeavouring to influence your body's ability to adapt for the challenges it faces from day to day. Whether we have a specific sporting career or are just on the treadmill of life, we ask an awful lot of ourselves, and refinement is the key to our self-management. In turn, becoming aware of the consequences of our lifestyle movement choices will facilitate the ability to make more informed decisions on what movement modalities to include that work best for each one of us. Quiet, simple, and subtle movement is actually a long-forgotten skill that has been lost to the pursuit of goal-oriented performance. While precision is something we might take for granted as young people, it can become elusive as we mature if there is no understanding of how it needs to be honoured and refined.

Myofascial magic in action will first make you fully conscious of your natural abilities and consciously distinguish limitations. As you learn about the structural influences your movement choice has on your internal architecture, the better and more eloquent decisions you will naturally make to refine your control over how your body moves and functions in variable motion. What is considered is:

1. Appropriate positioning
2. Precise sequencing
3. Effortless energy
4. Moving deliberately and deliciously

Our approach is to focus on efficiency of motion through confident transitions. The art of movement is to enhance your awareness of how you are interacting with your environment. Then movement choices can be consciously made to naturally re-educate the *unconscious* control. It hones movement as a skill and the intuitive and instinctive practices of organizing appropriately for the day, the time, and the event we find ourselves in.

Thereby, a skill is born! (A skill we can keep once we know how we attained it.) To this end, we focus on creating challenging environments via the use of many variations and specific props. These ensure you are fully present and engaged in the choice of positioning. That precedes the sequencing which in turn facilitates the intensity you can manage without compromising your myofascial integrity. Therein lies the magic! With that level of kindness, awareness, and astute game-raising with yourself, the body naturally gives back its best performance!

THE KEYSTONE

Muscles do not contract – muscles tension fascia.

(Jaap van der Wal)[41]

This is a quote from Jaap van der Wal that underpins why I believe *refine* is the keystone to understanding how we move at our best and restore our natural patterns optimally. It's a relationship made in harmony with the structure, the fabric, and the form of the body. In other words, whatever shape we are in, we can find harmony and refine our movements as a self-perpetuating advantage.

Traditional academic education bases movement on muscular contractions. It generally informs us that this process happens in isolation, via a particular muscle attached to a particular bone, which then provides an appropriate force to move a joint, thus creating the desired motion.

This is the bedrock theory of the musculo-skeletal system, backed up by the sliding filament theory which is another familiar explanation in human motion. This understanding misses out a most important ingredient and essential element of the story. If there is a muscle-spindle, then, given that there is no such thing as 'muscle' without the fascia in which it forms and arises, there *must* then be a corresponding fascial (environmental) spindle at the same location.

WHERE IS YOUR FASCIA?

Fascia is the most ubiquitous tissue within your whole body. It forms the environment of every cell and tissue. It forms the environment that every system exists and behaves within, having a plethora of roles to perform and interact amongst a symphony of co-existing systems. Besides its many influential roles (given that books on neurology and biomechanics are being rewritten), fascia's *relationship* with the neurological system, must be emphasized with its intertwined muscular system, without which neither (muscle nor nerve) could exist or function.

---

41   van der Wal, J. (2022) Presentation at Kings College London Anatomy Dissection Laboratory.

As muscles (appear to) 'shorten' or 'lengthen', they are in a corresponding relationship that tensions the surrounding fascial environment within which each muscle sarcomere lives. By this tensioning effect, a dynamic reaction occurs that enables structural integrity to be achieved and efficient motion to commence. No one can move via contraction of one without the other; they cannot be separated. Nor can they be relegated to one specific site (i.e., within the muscle) without a corresponding tensioning of the neighbouring structures, i.e., other muscles, skin, or bone and cartilage and ligament. All these aspects of so-called 'joints' are in complete continuity with the surrounding tissues, the entire length of the body.

Ligament isn't separate to bone, or the cartilage it invests. In few cases in the body does it only connect bone to bone without being invested in the cartilage surrounding the bones. It is in complete continuity within the wholeness of what is called a 'joint'. As such, Jaap van der Wal suggests (and provides excellent argument for) the naming of these points in our movement system as 'dynaments' (rather than ligaments) especially as they are in complete continuity with the whole.

Effectively, this tensioning (to appropriate frequency for the movement in question), is constantly tuning forces and their transmission *through* the dynamic structure in motion. This harmonic relationship is called a dynament (dynamic ligament tensioning) and must work seamlessly for effortless transfer of power and the associated forces to be distributed appropriately throughout the body. It almost acts like a volume control on the force transmission. When refined and balanced, it sounds like the best harmony the orchestra can participate in together. What that means is that for every move we make, there is a counterbalancing non-moving that requires similar attention. We orchestrate the smallest move throughout the body – even including what is in stillness.

Unfortunately, training in general is based on twentieth-century anatomy that describes every part of the body as a separate item and treats the musculo-skeletal system separately from the nervous system, attributing motion to nerves firing muscles to move bones. The general focus on strengthening and stretching the 'red muscle elements' in the anatomy atlas, without understanding the dramatic and dynamic effects on the 'white architectural fabric' comes at a cost. That fabric dictates the form, the ability to adapt, to refine and to facilitate optimum function. It's called the fascia matrix and it changes how we view movement and optimize it!

Understanding the consequences of ignoring (and even abusing) this simultaneously robust and delicate fabric is paramount to understanding movement for longevity and purpose.

If the fascia's ability to adapt and develop in a way that ensures gliding qualities is compromised, then the result will be a loss in sensory feedback. Gliding must be *consistently* maintained within the extracellular matrix. That is an essential enhancement of refined movement, and inhibition will be the main outcome if tissue glide is suboptimal. The body will naturally do that (inhibit movement) to protect itself. It is also essential that fascia is not over tensioned by excessive muscular forces (such as over training in the gym) as fascia thickens under extreme tensional forces, designed to resist tissue tearing.

Its fasciategral structure fundamentally resists deformation in all directions. Such a situation then makes the environment and structural location less mobile, or even immobilizes it if inflammation results, which can invite damage and subsequent pathology. With the new knowledge (the true knowledge) of fascia available, it is wise to be thoughtful about the choice of movement modalities and functional training methods. Extremes of strength training can often inadvertently create a dysfunctional outcome. Myofascial magic lives in the knowledge that muscle tensions fascia!

STRETCHING

The last section in this beautiful journey of refinement is to ask if living tissue is designed to be stretched. If I answer that question by saying, 'Absolutely not, the living human architectural matrix is an anti-stretching tissue *designed* to stop you falling. We need to respect its natural boundaries and constraints and not exceed them', would this confuse your current understanding of stretching?

Is living tissue designed to stretch? Think about that for a moment as you sit in your chair reading this. Are you returning from work or are you about to have dinner? Are you going training? What is your current interpretation of stretching? How does stretching benefit you and how often are you instructed to stretch or feel the need to?

As humans we have created a society and lifestyle that separates us from the world of nature; everything 'civilized' around us is generally manmade, linear, hard, and contained. Is it any wonder we want to push the boundaries of what our bodies can do and achieve, in the fleeting time we are able to do so?

We are, ourselves, very much part of nature; we are not mechanical, we do not move mechanically, and yet our whole healthcare, the fitness industry, and our life education around anatomy and physiology is based upon mechanics. This is not only misleading but reinforces the notion that we are separate from nature, rather than an integral species. If only we would return to our sense of connection, how different might our views and opinions be?

In the living world, all species are designed to survive and thrive within their respective environments. They do this in a sensory and reactive way, not just after the fact, but in anticipation and in a very highly tuned response to everything happening inside and out. All motion is fundamentally designed to be purposeful and graceful, to achieve maximum longevity with minimal inhibition of the functionality within the collective.

As an organic species ourselves, it only makes sense that our survival and ability to react in a timely and appropriate fashion during motion is directly reflective of nature's laws. That is not manmade laws of mechanics that, we are currently taught, *control us.*

So why do we stretch? What does it mean to be 'tight'? Why does it feel so good, and if it feels good and it's a pleasurable experience, how can that not be beneficial? These are very valid questions and require an appropriate response.

Let's look at life experiences, where our body reacts to stretching in a very natural way. Childbirth: if the results of stretching were what we aim for, babies would fall out of the birth canal and there would be no obstacle to our entering into the world. (See Recoil, by Dr Karen Kirkness, for more on this marvellous feature of the human body).

How about going for a walk and unexpectedly tripping on uneven ground? If it was unexpected and you were not able to anticipate this change of environment (i.e., the ground being uneven or cracked) your body momentarily behaved as if it was out of control as it trips. What your body does *not* do automatically is go into the 'splits' or do double somersaults at full length, like a gymnast. What actually happens, *immediately the sense of control goes*, is the body *decelerates* quickly to avoid falling; you instinctively seek to regain balance and the body does this by reacting quickly to *shorten* its living tissues, not lengthen them. It tries to protect you as it activates its anti-stretching characteristics to limit the damage of falling.

In martial arts, one of the most prolific styles is ju-jitsu. The whole essence of ju-jitsu is to contain and inhibit another person's ability to move, and to threaten the boundaries of the limbs, neck, and spine in such a way that the opponent submits to the threat of being taken beyond their natural protective boundaries. However, if stretching were appropriate, we would never submit, but allow our bodies to keep stretching. We would enjoy and embrace the experience of our body being taken to such extremes. We don't because we are instinctively threatened by it.

Let us consider the gymnasts, dancers, yogis and martial artists whose whole methodologies and training regimes are focused on stretching the living tissue beyond its natural boundaries and constraints, that the sensory fascia and neurological system provides. I have met hundreds of these practitioners after decades of this apparently 'appropriate approach', who explain to me how they now have to manage the consequences and ramifications of those training protocols. They now deal with daily pain, pathologies, and even surgical interventions, as a result of having pushed their bodies beyond physical capabilities, and taken away the structural constraints overriding the natural defences. Those training protocols should help them succeed within their given discipline, not predispose their bodies to fail in the face of practicing it.

What I have found, from my experience of working for over 20 years in all these movement disciplines, is that generally, teachers believe they are stretching the red muscular fibres in the anatomy atlas to help hydrate the tissue. In fact, they are challenging the fascial, architectural tissues (the white tissue in the atlas) and its immediate environment. These red muscular fibres inhabit the architectural fabric of the entire body's natural sensory defensive system. It is virtually the 'environmental responsibility' of the sensory receptors at the folds in the tissue structures, to maintain, manage, and react in a timely fashion, to resist deformation. As such, they resist when stretch effects are placed upon them.

What this means is that you are not stretching muscles. The stretching is actually being forced through the neuromyofascial system. That includes the neurological tissues and the other vessels of the body. Nothing gets left out of this body-wide communication network.

Be careful! For every neurological initiation, there is a chemical reaction to facilitate motion. That means that as you 'stretch your neurology' you could be challenging the chemistry in an inappropriate way. This then affects the balance of chemical reactions that should occur for efficiency and longevity. In turn, this can often create an energy crisis within the myofascial environment, commonly creating something known as myofascial trigger points. They hurt.

These formations of chemical bonding within the myofascial tissues do not only have an influence on movement, but also on the general ability to live freely; in terms of motion and being pain free. All athletes, who take their bodies to extreme measures, shorten their time in their chosen sport. Although we all strive to enjoy life and make the most of the opportunities it gives us, taking on challenges that really push us beyond our boundaries, even in the most positive way, are not always as beneficial to our long-term health.

There is always a price to pay, and your living tissue will pay it every day. Understand that adaptation is not limitless in the negative form; negative adaptation to movement has a threshold, and once you reach that threshold, injury, pathology, and surgery will likely follow. However, positive adaptation is limitless if you are respecting your living tissues' boundaries and respecting your living tissues' ability to thrive within their local and global environments. True longevity of the one living structure you will ever have control over, without ever requiring attention of the healthcare or fitness industries, must be our true aspiration.

But what about the pleasurable side of stretching? Why does it feel so good?

Let us understand that our body's only requirement is to survive and resist threat to itself. Regardless of what we perceive to be threatening our life, what that means is that tissue (at its subconscious instinctive level) is primarily efficient. It utilizes its two options:

1. It can shorten and stiffen, which we often interpret as 'tightening'. This is a restrictive measure that inhibits movement options. It is actually a protective response, which we can often override by trying to stretch tissue that is trying to stop us moving! It has an innate intelligence, designed to prevent the damage of stretching.

2. If the tightening response above is ineffective and *does not prevent you overriding your own self defence mechanisms*, it will do the

opposite and go passive. This is not a good thing, that has a yogi thinking, 'Oh great, I've finally managed to do the splits.' This is going beyond physiological range; the tissue takes this extreme by releasing a chemical called endocannabinoid. Like cannabis, it's a relaxant and a pleasurable experience in the short term.

In movement, this can make you go passive and dormant, another protective mechanism to the threat of the movement you are putting it through, which it considers beyond range. This is often misinterpreted as improving your range of movement when all you have achieved is reducing your ability to move optimally and react appropriately during active motion. That tissue can't restore anymore because you have damaged its ability to return within physiological range. You have effectively overridden a natural defensive reflex and the long-term cost of that is joint laxity and subsequently pain. It is the opposite of short-term pain for long-term gain. It is short-term pain-release for long-term loss of structural integrity.

In mediaeval times, people were put on 'the rack' to interrogate them and obtain information against their will. The most painful form of punishment was to be 'hung, drawn and quartered'. It was effectively stretching the body to tearing point, beyond any attempt of the body to produce the chemicals that soothe injury in the short term. Now we willingly place ourselves within the rack to experience it, the pleasure of stretching, for the euphoric feelings that result. The long-term price is high.

The kind of stretching we do when we yawn and stretch is very different in quality and intention from the intensive stretching that, for some unknown reason, has become a pre-requisite of many movement modalities. When yawning, the muscles *decelerate* and squeeze the tissues at the same time as lengthening them. It self-protects the relentless nature of just 'pulling' and allows for a natural reset. It is also designed as an after-rest reset, *not* a 'pre-performance preparation'. Watch any wild cat (or domestic one at that). They will stretch and yawn when they get up from resting. You will never see one preparing to hunt, by stretching. They shorten and tighten the tissue, from the hair follicles on the back of their necks, and whiskers, down to their claws – they tighten everything to spring-load their bodies to pounce.

Animals never take their bodies beyond physiological (fasciategral) range for pleasure. The misguided sense of euphoria comes with the body's natural protective system that will help reduce pain when a tear or injury takes place. It is very common after damaging a ligament or breaking a bone that the body doesn't begin to feel high intensity pain until afterwards. That isn't a license to lengthen the tissue more. It is a nature-given feature designed to give us time to get out of trouble and protect ourselves from further danger or threat.

The adage 'just move it or lose it' is not only inappropriate but reflects poorly on a fitness industry that is constantly having to deal with the consequences of moving poorly. It is something like saying 'just play the guitar' to someone who has no clue how to tune it, how to hold it, position themselves correctly, or play a chord properly. They have to acquire those different skills before achieving the skilful ability to play a song that is in tune!

It seems that despite all of us living inside it, we know little about the human form, even though what we do know is awesome. We are far removed from moving only as a musculo-skeletal body. Learning how different assets and aspects of motion (like the guitarist in the example above) affect our living tissues, helps us to inform ourselves of how to refine our movements and manage the ramifications of our choices. Not all movement is optimal!

Movement is skilled, otherwise anyone could do it and nobody would ever get injured. What I call 'longevity of choice' is the crown jewel of our species, but we focus so much on intensity that it shortens our ability to attain the longevity of choice we seek.

Movement is not medicine if it is done poorly; movement is a skill long forgotten and we take for granted the refinement that actually needs to be learned and practiced. Remember rebound, recoil, release, restore, and refine! The more you refine, the less you will need to practice the others; they will come naturally!

PRACTICE SECTION: THE FIVE Rs

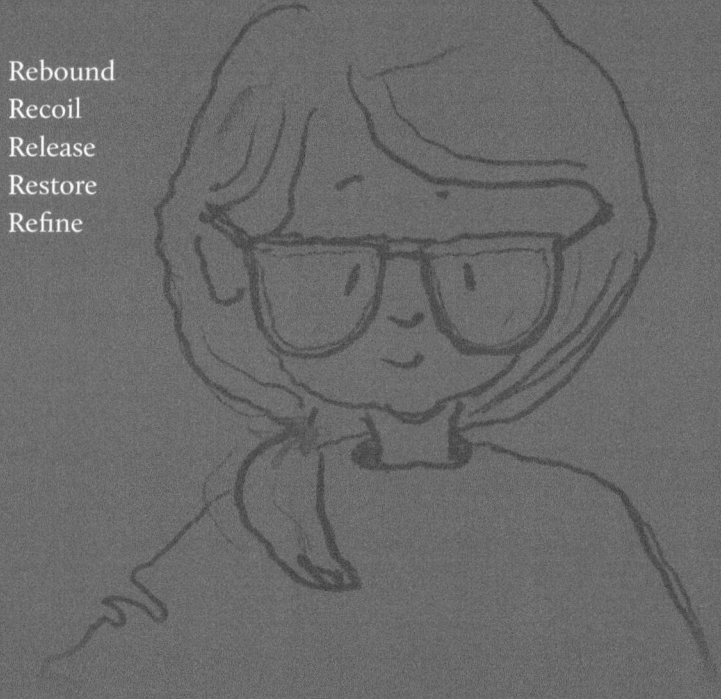

PROPS REQUIRED

Soft ball and resistance band

Throughout the sequences, the props required are a **low resistance band** and one or two **soft stability balls**. Both are readily available online.

The resistance band (lowest is best at around 5 kg resistance) is approximately 2 metres in length. You then learn to 'feel' how you (or your client) needs to hold the band for the right tension. (These can be bought on a roll and cut to size).

Soft stability balls: (Resistance can be changed with how much they are inflated). You can play with different sizes – 7, 9, or 12 inch – using them at various levels of inflation depending on the moves. It is useful to have at least two – one to support the head (more deflated) and one to do the movements (more inflated).

PRACTICE SECTION 1: REBOUND

Rebound 1: finding the frame

Purpose: Learning patterns of integrity when we change direction, tempo, height, and orientation within our environment, to cultivate stability and the ability to control the outcome of our movement choices. Complete a few repetitions of each variation before doing the final version.

Support: In your standing ground print make sure that your feet are comfortably spaced to support you. The compressive effect of the ball creates a light tensional reaction throughout your structure. This proprioceptive feedback invites you to notice how the framework you've created supports your motion and helps you to maintain structural integrity as you add more variables to the movements.

Timing: The essence of timing in these exercises is to find rhythmic motion as weight transfers over the base or ground print. Explore the temporal quality of acceleration and deceleration whilst maintaining competency to react and adapt to the motions in a timely fashion.

Sequence:

▶ Interlacing the fingers, place and lightly compress the stability ball against the chest, whilst equally pressing the chest into the ball, establishing proprioceptive awareness of the frame.

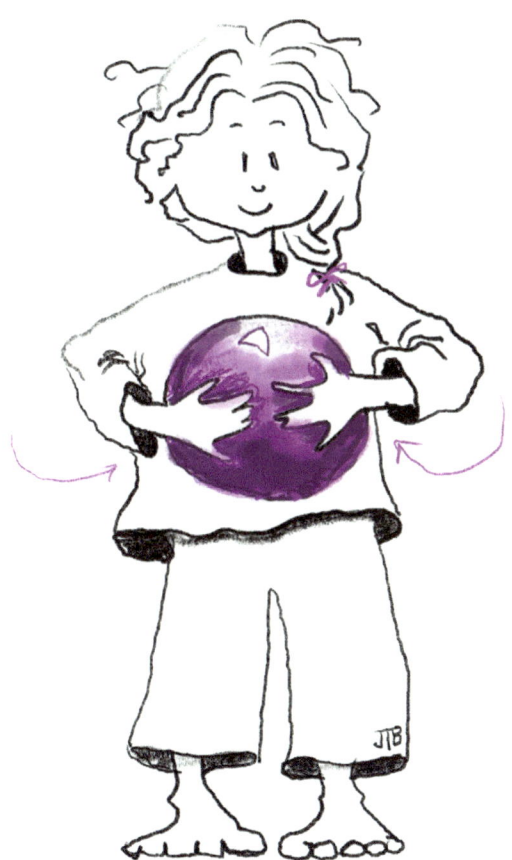

Figure 42 Rebound 1.1.

▸ Circle the shoulders, making sure the shoulder blades are free to glide on the back of the ribs (Figure 43), then gently rotate the torso towards the left and then the right, finding the natural 'central' position of the ribcage turning gently over the pelvis (Figure 44).

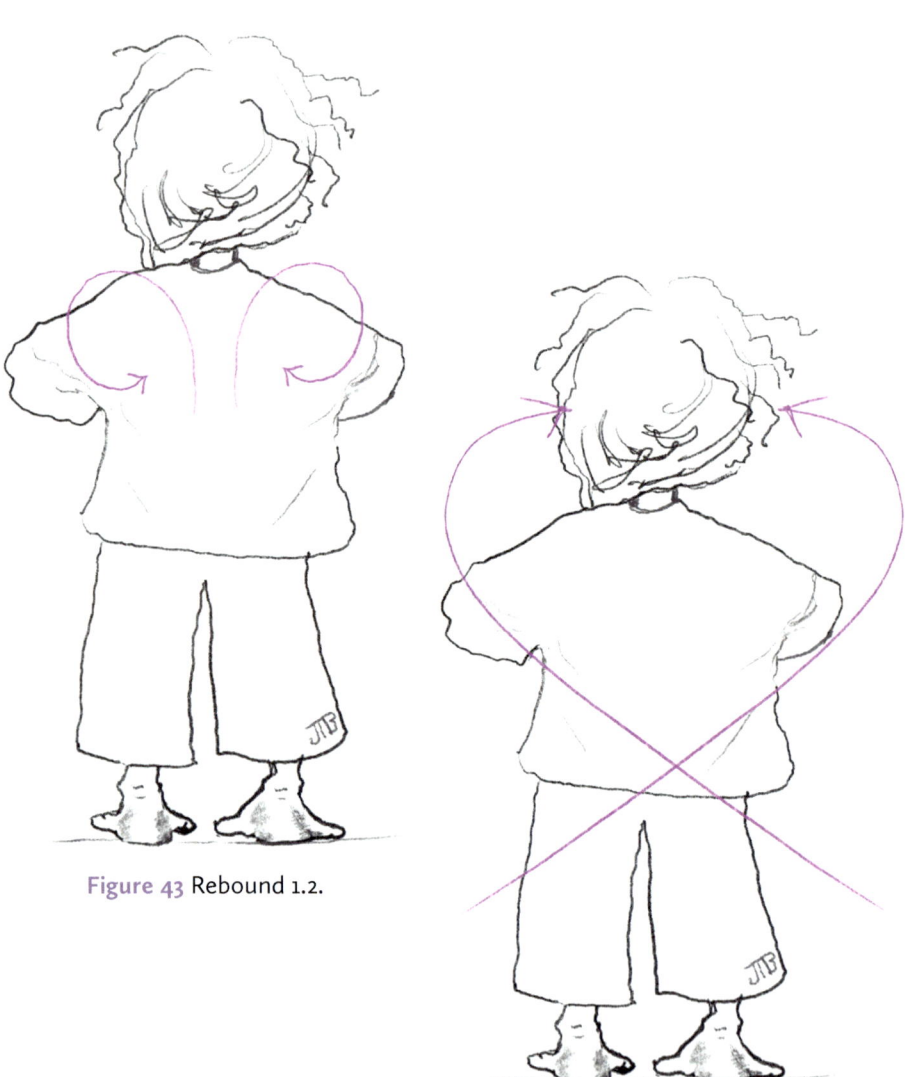

Figure 43 Rebound 1.2.

Figure 44 Rebound 1.3.

▶ Raise the heels up and down, rising and descending without deviating from the integral shape that's already been created with the ball against the chest. Do this a few times to establish a rhythm.

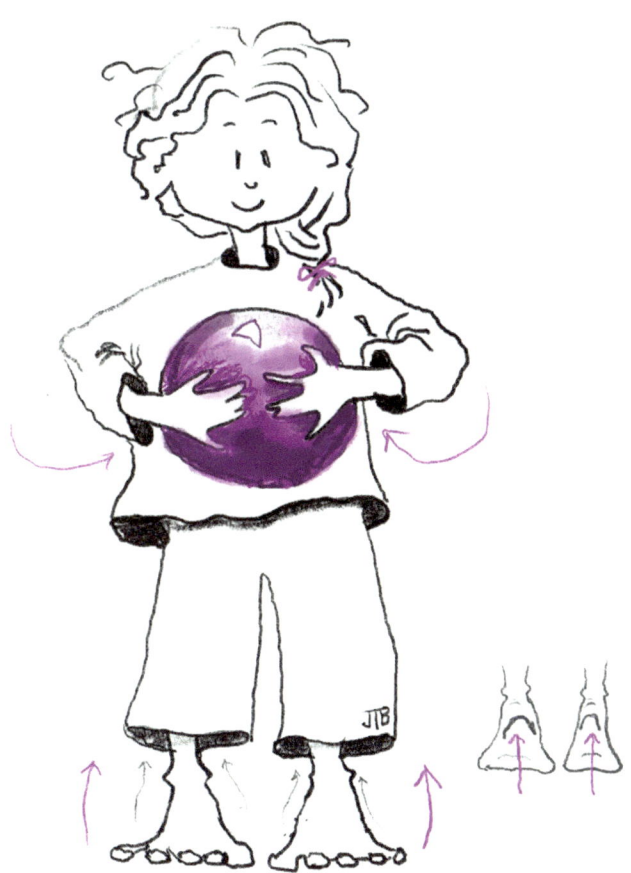

Figure 45 Rebound 1.4.

▸ *Variation 1:* Stagger the feet by taking one step forward. Rock forward bringing the heels off the ground, transferring the weight back, then bringing the toes off the ground. (Repeat with the other foot forward.)

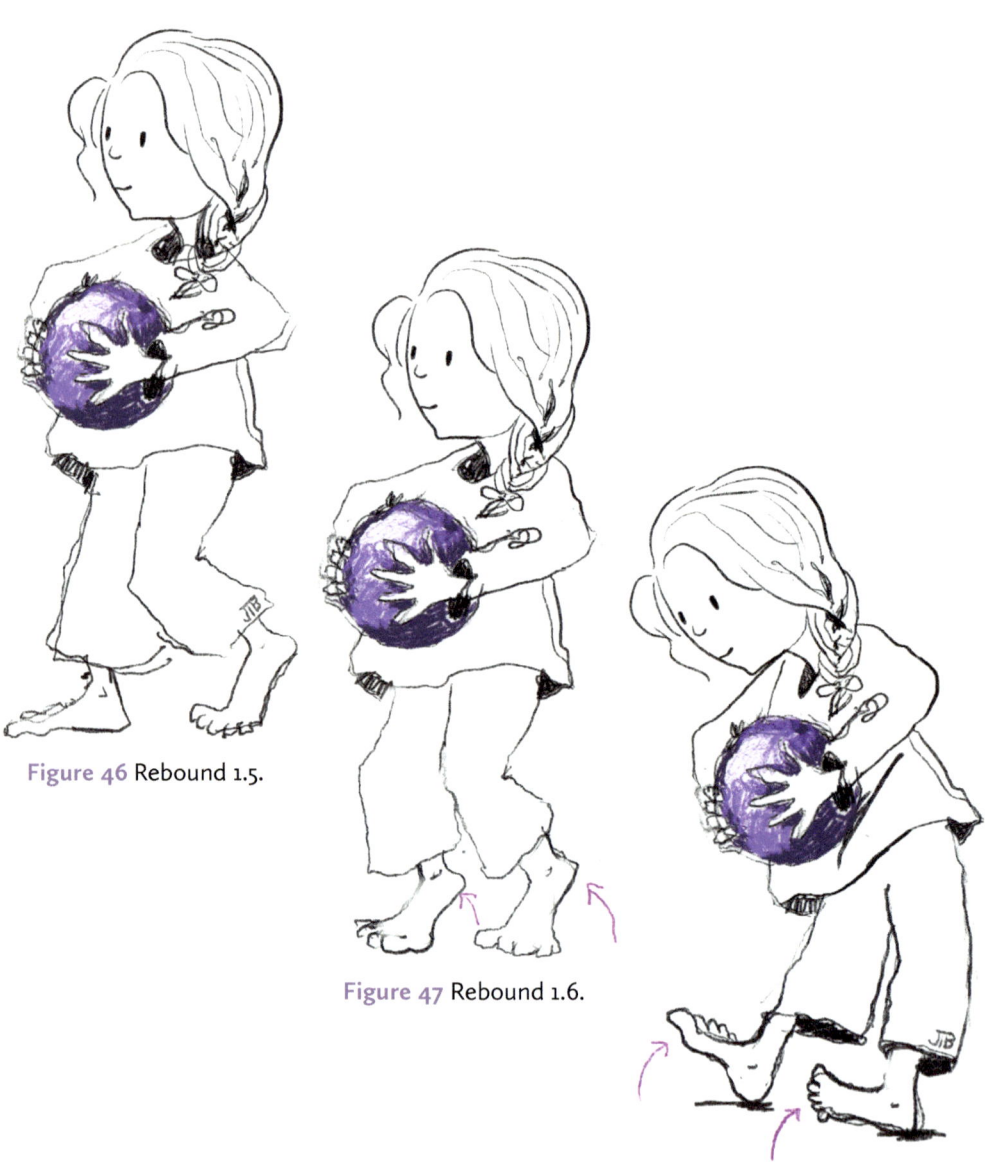

Figure 46 Rebound 1.5.

Figure 47 Rebound 1.6.

Figure 48 Rebound 1.7.

▸ *Variation 2:* Now take two steps forward, then two steps back, finding rhythm to the movement. Maintaining the integrity of the ball, lightly against the chest. Go lightly through the feet, back and forth. (Repeat taking two steps forward, then two steps back, starting with the other foot.)

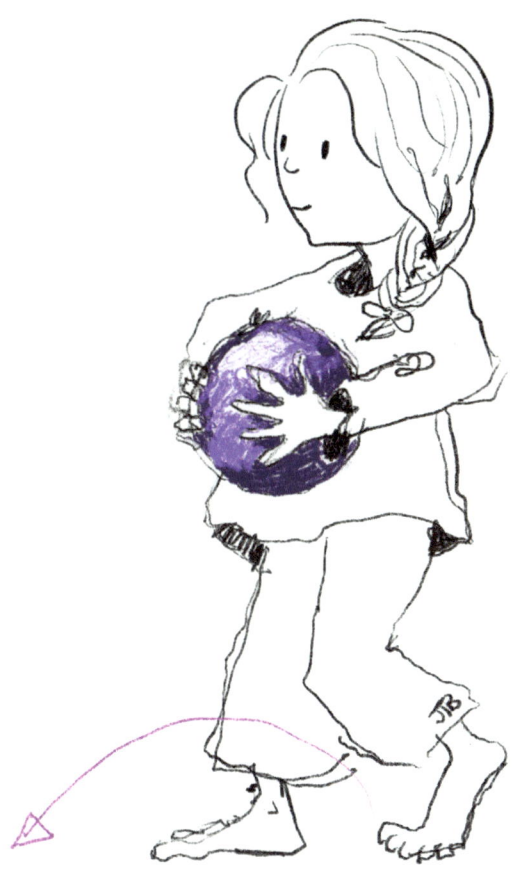

Figure 49 Rebound 1.8.

▶ *Variation 3:* Return to the staggered ground print (Variation 1) by taking one step forward. Find the rhythmic rocking pattern, moving forward and back. As the heels are raised off the ground, push the knees forward to lower the body towards the ground *gently decelerating* as far as is comfortable. Make sure the *back heel* is as high as possible as the knees fold. To come back to vertical, find the somasense of *pulling the knees up* rather than pushing up from the feet. (Repeat with the other foot forward.)

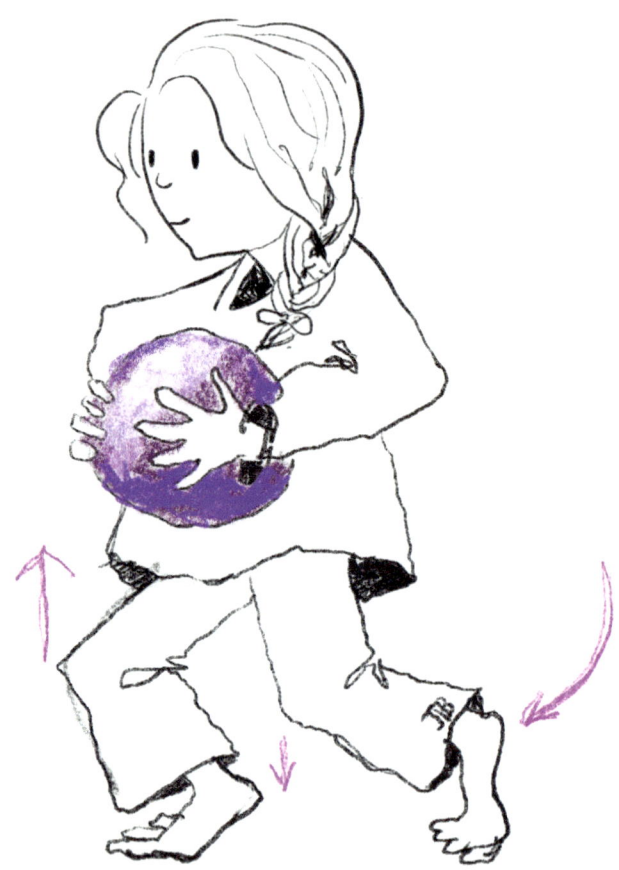

Figure 50 Rebound 1.9.

▸ Myofascial magic moment: Now explore the same sequence of move-ments without the ball, paying close attention to the frame and body organization. Experience the difference with and without the ball. Over time, with practice, the same biomotional integrity will become available with and without the ball.

▸ *Practitioner note: It can help to do each variation with and without the ball, so that the body-wide sensory awareness can be somatically awakened to the subtle differences in proprioceptive awareness. This is essentially what is being animated and gradually, over time, sustained as a resource within the body. It becomes familiar with the 'frame' and structurally sustaining postural integrity naturally.*

Rebound 2: finding deeper rebound

Purpose: Changing the floor, the environment the body walks on, changes proprioceptive awareness. Adding endurance brings the capacity to move freely. The floor changes everything and, in the natural world, changes all the time.

Support: Use the support of a wall or chair if needed for this balancing exploration. Make sure that the foot on the ball is placed directly under-neath the knee to optimize the rebound motion.

Timing: As the foot bounces on the ball, seek to establish a continuous steady rhythm. The rhythm is optimal, so use a chair or wall for support to find the rhythm, then seek to maintain it without the support (if appropriate) once the body can maintain rhythmical balance. The focus is primarily on a steady rhythm rather than on the balancing, so use sup-port until ease and competency is reached and can be easily maintained.

Sequence:

▸ With the feet in a staggered position, place the stability ball underneath the front foot. Make sure the foot is broad on the ball, and there is no grabbing with the toes. Raise the heel to midway, slightly off the ball, so it has the ability to move up and down (rebound) as necessary.

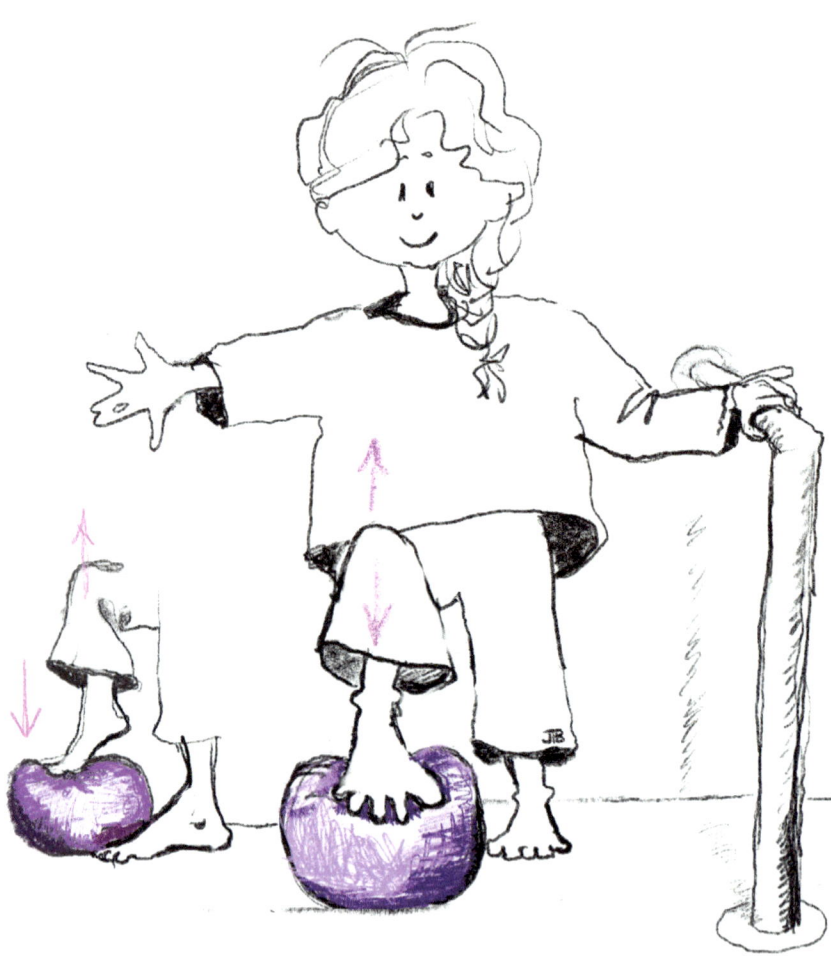

Figure 51 Rebound 2.1.

▶ Re-establish the frame and vertical organization of the body, with the toes of the standing leg broad on the mat or floor, not hooking the ground. (Use the wall or a chair or barre at first for support if required.) Start to bounce the foot on the ball, creating a rebound effect, barely lifting the toes from the surface of the ball. Find a rhythm and repeat while integrity is maintained in the movement and the upright position. Repeat on the other side.

The supporting leg, meanwhile, is working, too. It is improving its relationship with the torso, and overall shape from ground to crown. Don't collapse into the standing hip. Notice how this challenges both the ability to create rhythmical rebound *and* the ability to maintain upright balance, as the supporting leg is holding the frame.

Rebound 3: finding micro-refine for macro-play

Purpose: Transferring weight forward and back whilst building endurance. This supports control as a resource for any rebounding activities, when the step changes while moving forward.

Support: Use the support of a wall or chair and make sure the body feels very supported in the long stride position with the front/forward knee facing in the same direction as the toes.

Timing: Explore quality of movement within a time frame. The focus is not repetition for repetition's sake. It is fine-tuning so that when there is occasion for more random movements (in a ball game, for example) the body is building in its ability to change direction swiftly, easily, and without disorientation.

Sequence:

▸ Take a long stride with the front leg facing forward, knee bent. The
back leg is long and lengthened with a sense of drawing the kneecap
up. Lift the back heel away from the ground, toes tucked under and
spread wide and comfortably.

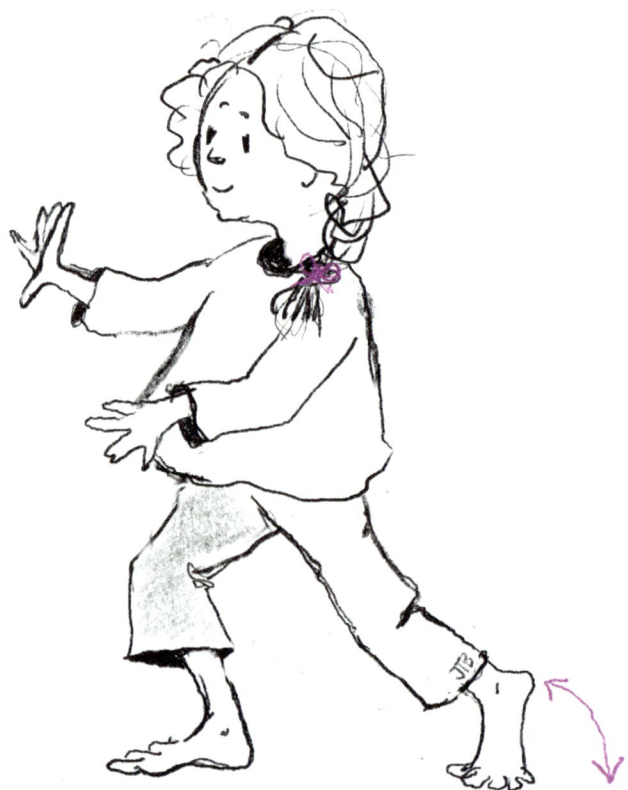

Figure 52 Rebound 3.1.

▸ Push forward, through the back foot, to transfer the weight over the
front leg, and initiate coming back by a pull through the back foot.
Transfer the weight forward and back, finding a rhythmic pattern
(pulling from the back heel, rather than pushing from the front knee).
Keep both feet in contact with the floor.

▸ *Variation 1:* From the long stride position, push through the back foot this time with a little more effort, transferring the weight fully through the front leg so that *the back foot floats effortlessly off the ground*. Position the hands as though they are gently pushing the space in front of the body away, to help support the balance as the weight is transferred to the front foot. (This is not jumping – it is a progression to the back foot floating.)

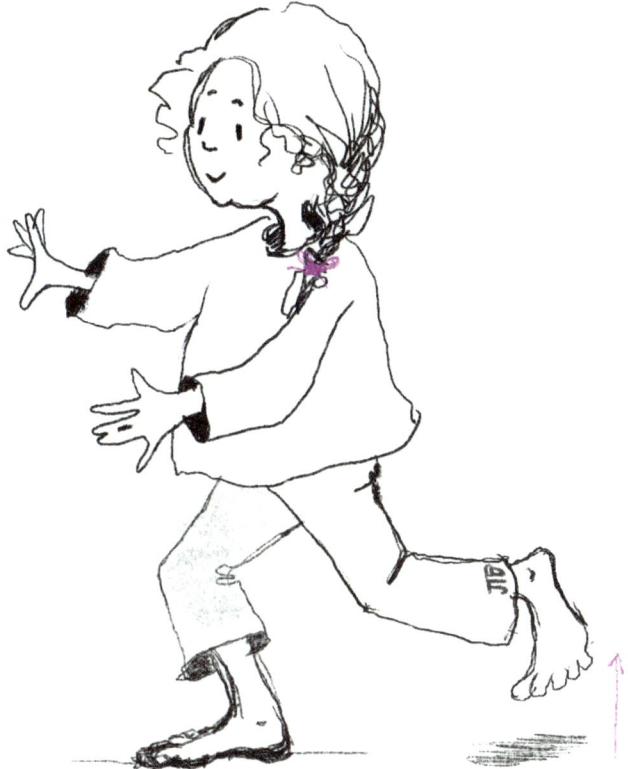

Figure 53 Rebound 3.2.

▸ Glide the back foot back towards the ground and continue to repeat the movement, exploring the quality of the full forward-return movement within a comfortable timeframe. (Do not force a number of repetitions. Rather find the movement integrity, even if one or two is the maximum that can be done with ease).

▸ *Practitioner note: 'Ease' is denoted by an effortless ability to lift the back foot off the ground and place it back on the return motion, with quiet control.*

▸ *Variation 2:* This time, as all the weight is transferred to the front leg, make sure the front leg is happy to take the load and gradually bring the back leg forward through space, by bending the knee, bringing it in front of the torso, then taking it back. Repeat the movement exploring the quality of the motion.

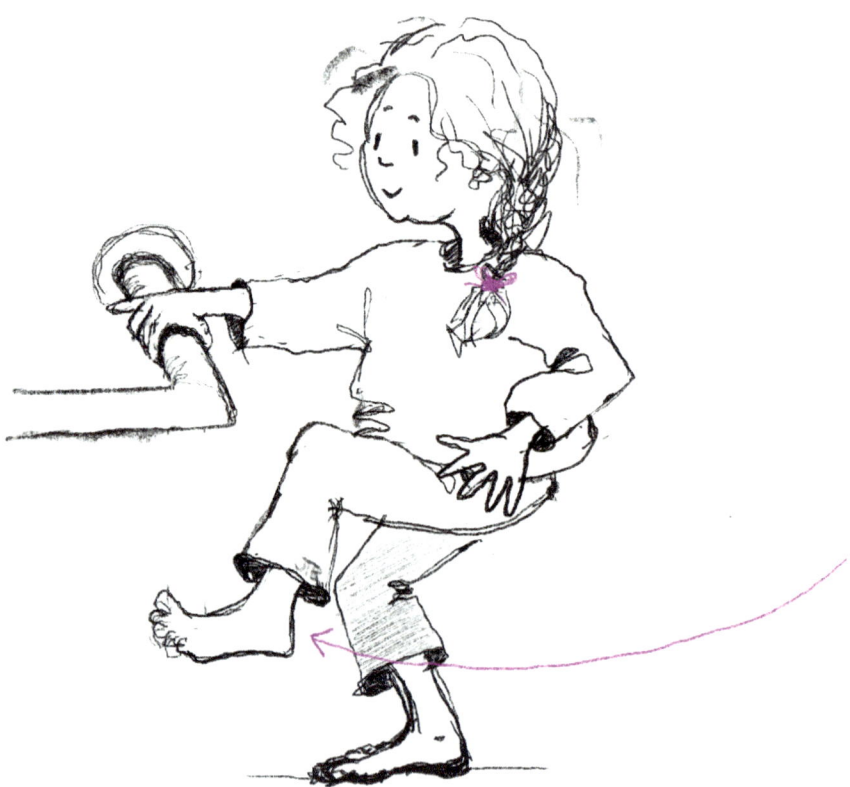

Figure 54 Rebound 3.3.

▸ **Modification:** If required, hold a chair, barre, or wall for support. This is usually most helpful on the side of the back leg, supporting moving it forward. If the above movements are too intense for the *front* leg, a low intensity moderation is to draw the back leg forward while keeping the toes on the floor, gliding along the ground. As the weight is transferred back, for the return motion, keep the back heel raised from the ground. (Wearing socks on a smooth floor helps this one, but *only* if it is health and safety appropriate for the practice environment. It is worth exploring as it builds in versatility as an asset.)

PRACTICE SECTION 2: RECOIL

Recoil 1: standing where folds counter rotate

Purpose: This is about exploring natural constraint patterns, and intentional constraint of certain default movement patterns to experience (and enhance) the innate recoil capacity of the individual myofascial matrix. This is an inquiry into how energy is directed through the structure for different purposes: creating living fasciategral response exploring turning and spiralling recoil.

Support: Standing exploration. If working with a client, ask their permission to provide them with sensory feedback placing hands on the side of their pelvis, ribs, and head at the appropriate points.

Timing: Explore each side of the rotational movements with the intention to sense the quality of motion. This is an explorative sensory inquiry, which can be experimented with over time to notice if there are any changes to the quality of the movements.

Sequence:

▸ This sequence is an excellent 'soft assessment tool' for working with clients, as well as using personally to identify patterns and biases within one's own movements.

▸ Torso rotation: Standing with arms by the sides or crossed and resting on the chest, begin rotating. Observe inwardly, sensing the quality of the movement as the rotations turn towards the right and then the left. Self-assess (or client assess) asking, 'How does left and right rotation compare? Is there any restriction in the movement? How fluid does the motion feel?'

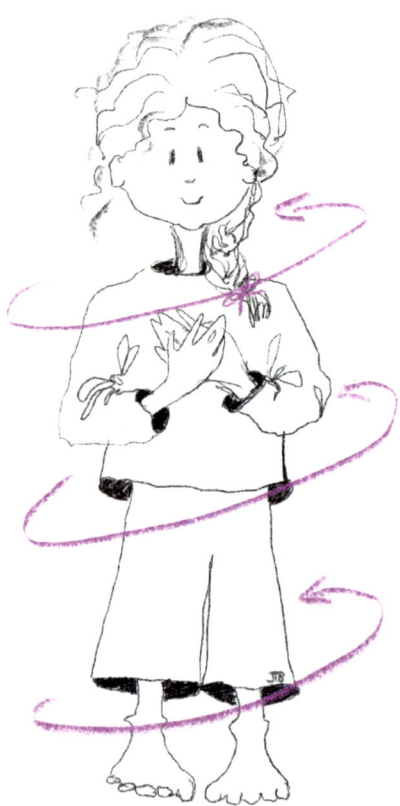

Figure 55 Recoil 1.1.

▶ *Practitioner note: There are no right or wrong answers; it is to establish difference and ease, or lack thereof. Please don't force this or do it too quickly. It is not goal oriented or 'how far is the rotation' as if further is better. It is simply to validate somasense of rotational compliance.*

▶ *Variation 1:* Counter rotation: As the pelvis rotates, notice if the rib basket can *counter* rotate. (This can be deceptive as it may be that the whole torso is moving as one, with little distinction between ribs and pelvis). For this variation, in self-assessment, constrain movement at the pelvis and rotate *only* the ribs to the left and then right sides. If client assessing, ask permission to place the hands on the sides of their pelvis to minimize movement (adding subtle constraint) whilst the client gently rotates their ribs only.

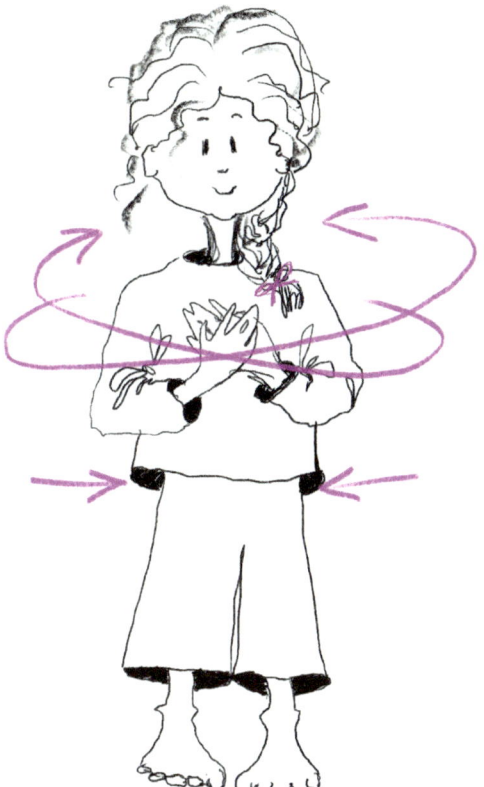

Figure 56 Recoil 1.2.

▶ Sense the ability and constraint in *counter rotation*. Notice if there are discrepancies between the left and right rotation of the ribs in counter rotation to the pelvis. Is one side more resistant or compliant than the other? If working with a client, listen with the hands to the *quality* of movement. Is there fluidity, resistance, or defensive reflexes within the motion? (These are examples; it becomes clear when there are differences from one side to the other). Don't force or overemphasize the differences; this is to sense change and progress over time.

▸ *Variation 2:* Continue to constrain movement at the pelvis whilst rotating the ribs, and this time make sure that movement in the neck and head is also gently constrained, so the only structure moving is the ribs. To help this in a subtle way, simply keep the eyes forward looking out to the horizon and the pelvis facing forward, while the ribs rotate in each direction. This is usually a very small, subtle movement.

▸ *Practitioner note: If permission is given, keep the hands gently on the side of the client's pelvis to keep it facing forward and encourage them to keep head facing (and eyes looking) forward.*

This gentle exploration can also be done in a seated pose. Sit up tall, with sitting bones on a cushion or ball, making sure the pelvis is 3 to 5 finger-widths higher than the knees when viewed from the side. This assists the natural spine curves which facilitate rotation.

Recoil 2: four-point kneeling; exploring hidden bias

Purpose: Experiencing rotational opportunities, knowing where the rotational biases are and directions that there is a tendency to favour or avoid. This improves inner self-awareness.

Support: Use the ground to receive sensory feedback through the whole structure.

Timing: Explore rotation and the opposing retraction and protraction of the shoulder blades as much as possible, whilst constraining the head and pelvis to generate counter-rotational forces. The key is to pay attention to shifts in the quality of the movement over time.

Sequence:

▸ Position the hands and knees on all fours on a comfortable surface. Place the hands slightly forward of the shoulders, as wide as necessary for comfort.

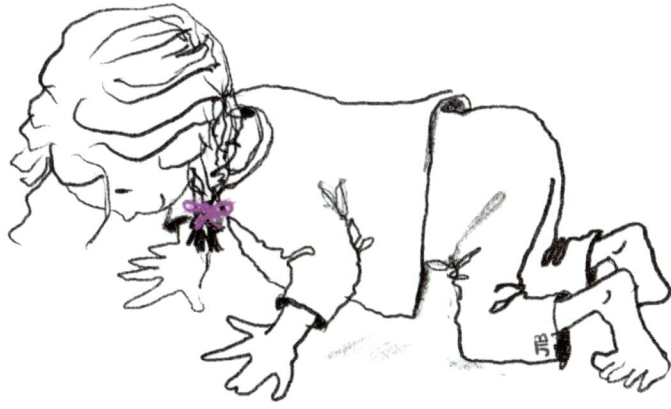

Figure 57 Recoil 2.1.

▶ Take one hand off the ground and place it on the same side at the upper thigh. This will enable the head, neck, shoulder, and thorax to rotate, as the shoulder blade retracts towards the spine. Constrain movement at the pelvis so it remains facing the floor.

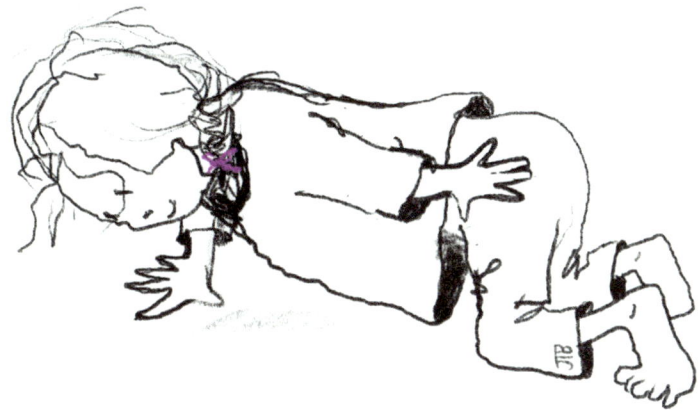

Figure 58 Recoil 2.2.

▶ Find a rhythm with this movement, sliding the hand up and down the thigh with each rotation. Use the breath to facilitate the movement, inhaling on the rise as the twist opens, exhaling on the descent, back to four-point kneeling position with torso parallel to floor. Then play with repeating the same movement, with the opposite breath pattern (exhaling on the rise and inhaling on the descent/return to parallel with the floor) and notice how it influences the movement. Do this breath practice on the other side.

▶ *Variation 1:* The next progression would be to rotate downwards protracting the shoulder blade, following the open rotation whilst keeping the head and pelvis still. Do this to both sides.

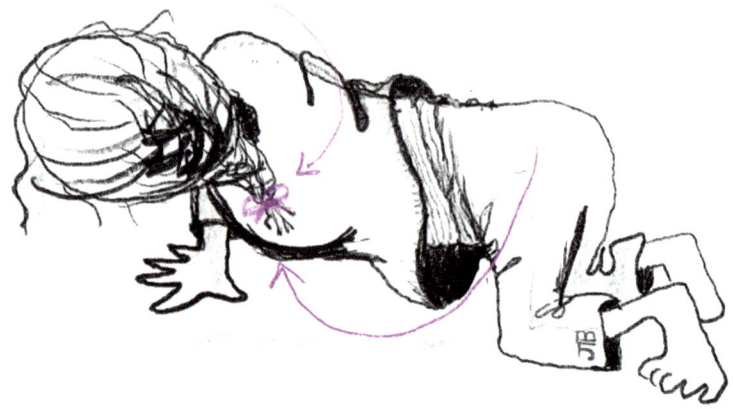

Figure 59 Recoil 2.3.

▶ *Variation 2:* Keep the pelvis and the eye-line facing the floor, with both hands to the floor. (If assisting a client, ask their permission to place subtle hands on either side of the head to gently help constrain movement.) Rotate the thorax only, keeping both the head and pelvis still, facing downward, to create a counter rotational effect. (Like the previous technique, this expresses as a small subtle movement.)

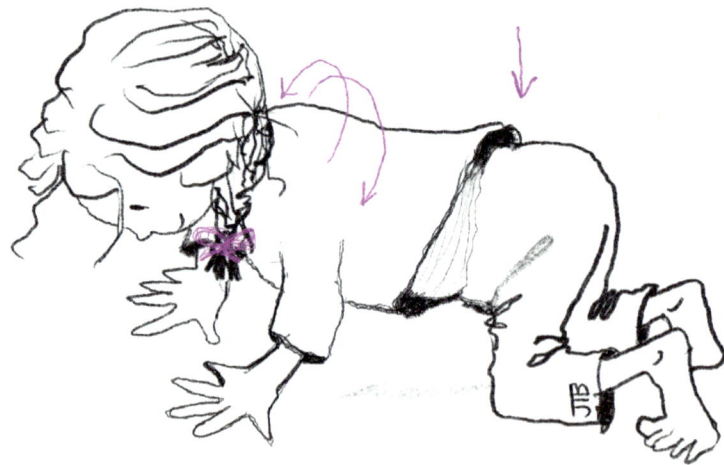

Figure 60 Recoil 2.4.

This set can be done kneeling, with hands against the wall, or using a barre in standing, if kneeling is inappropriate. In all cases, the emphasis is on sensing constraint and revealing (subtle) natural bias; it is rare that anyone has the same range to both sides. The subtle exploration encourages natural contralateral rotation in any activity or sport. This can be particularly valuable for racquet-players as they tend to play to a favoured side, swimmers with a bias towards their 'breathing' side, and parents tending to carry babies (or anyone carrying bags) on a favoured side to keep one hand free to do things. All these movements come at a price, costing the natural balance of contralateral freedom that this exercise is designed to support.

Recoil 3: spiral balances where we self-organize (using light resistance flexi band)

Purpose: All these practices feature learning and incorporating counter rotational forces. With that, it is possible to start to play more with endurance and intensity to help grow in competence and confidence in the body and movement choices.

Support: Light resistance flexi band, long enough to change the intensity of the resistance as required.

Timing: As the intensity builds, notice how long the movements can be done before feeling fatigued. The aim is to move as gracefully and fluidly as possible with the tensional support of the band. Don't think about repetition, think about the time frame. 'How long can this be done well and performed before tiring and before the quality starts to diminish?' Stop as soon as this sense of fatigue starts to happen, take a rest, and try again once (and if) there is energy to do so. With practice, this becomes easier and effortless, however, please avoid 'pushing to the limit' or the body will tend to avoid the movement, which is a super valuable resource to many everyday movements.

Sequence:

▸ Take the resistance band behind the back, holding it at each end with the hands. (The band goes underneath the armpits and over the inside of the upper arm. Hold it like a bunch of flowers, so you can easily adjust tension and keep it in place.) Reach the arms out to the side in a T position. Balance the intensity of the resistance band so that it's not too slack or pulled too tight (feel it 'just right' and not over tensioned – no strain across the hands, but enough tension to feel 'held' in the T position). Feel able to easily glide the scapula bones around whilst maintaining the appropriate tension of the band.

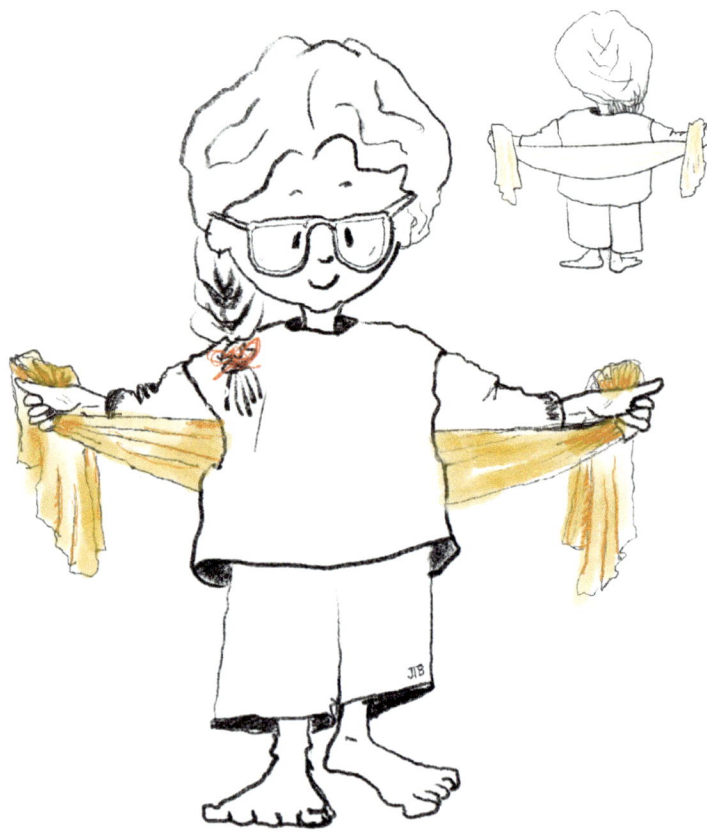

Figure 61 Recoil 3.1.

▶ Throughout this arm sequence, the original tension is maintained in the band. You'll notice you're creating a mobius or figure-eight movement through space by following the instructions.

▶ Keeping the arms out in the T position, choose which arm to move first. Turn the palm of that hand to face upwards to begin. Next, keeping the arm outstretched and the band tension in place, begin to reach that hand across the torso as if intending to *meet* the other hand (that stays out to the side) until the band prevents further movement. The first hand will naturally lift up slightly higher than the elbow and the palm will naturally begin to turn towards the floor just with the tension of the band.

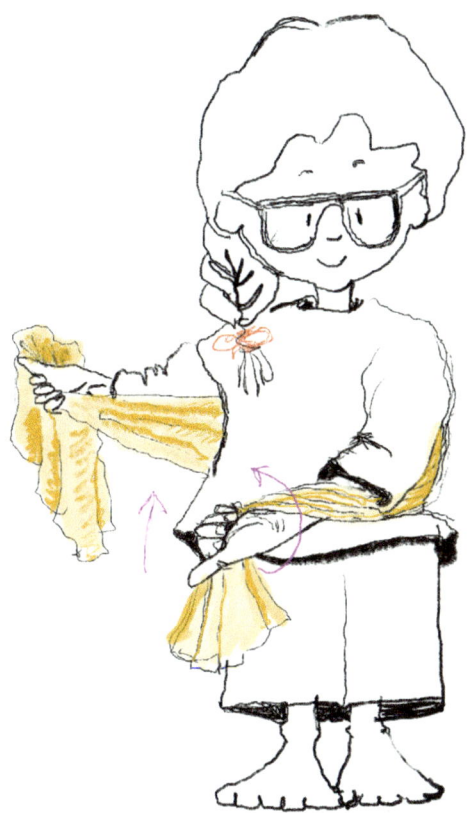

Figure 62 Recoil 3.2.

▸ Once the arm has come across to its end range (its natural fasciategral limit), turn the palm back up (again the hand will be higher than the elbow), then open it horizontally, taking the arm back out to the same side, in the starting position. Do this a few times, stopping if it is tiring.

▸ Try the sequence to the other side. Notice how the scapula bones move. Are they gliding with the motion being created by the rib-cage? Is the pelvis swaying and undulating with the movement or is it restricting the range? How are the feet responding to the ground? Is there a rhythm to the movement?

▸ *Variation 1:* Do this on one side, then the other in succession, feeling the rhythmical motion of making figure-eight shapes under tensional resistance; sensing the difference from one side to the other. (See Figure 63 to both sides; notice if one side feels 'easier' or 'smoother'.)

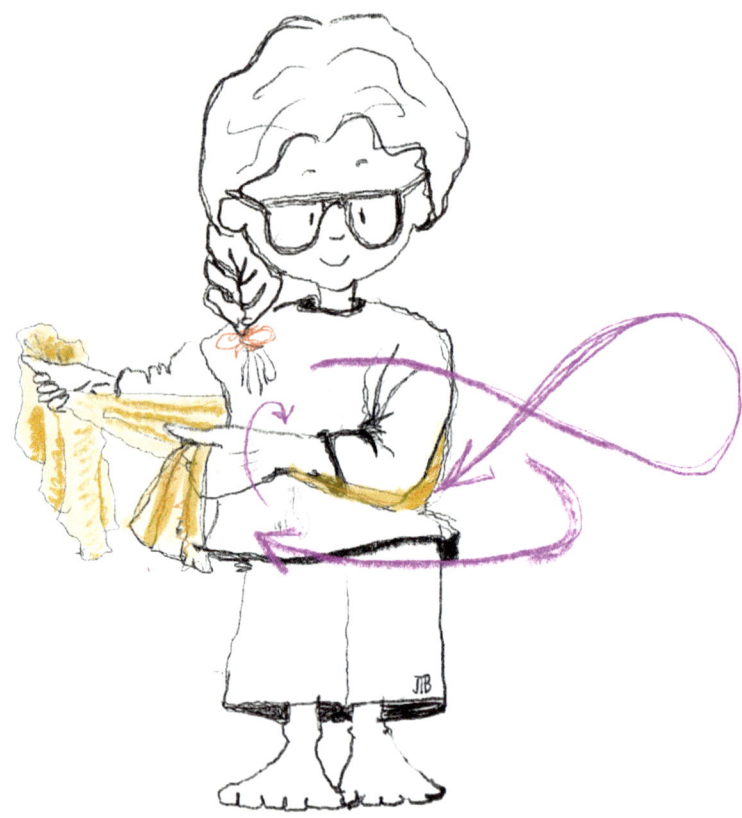

Figure 63 Recoil 3.3.

▸ *Variation 2:* The next progression from this is to add the legs to the movement. Maintaining the T position with the arms (don't move them in this variation), lunge one leg out to the side keeping the heel off the ground, immediately push off from the foot to bring the body back to the initial standing position. Repeat this movement to create a rebounding rhythm. Once there is confidence, explore changing the landing spot (in front, behind, and out to the side), maintaining the rhythmic rebound motion. Explore this on both legs. The lunge can begin very small, as a step to the side, and get bigger. Unpredictable movements, while maintaining the T position at the arms, increase the resilience and adaptability this is designed to promote.

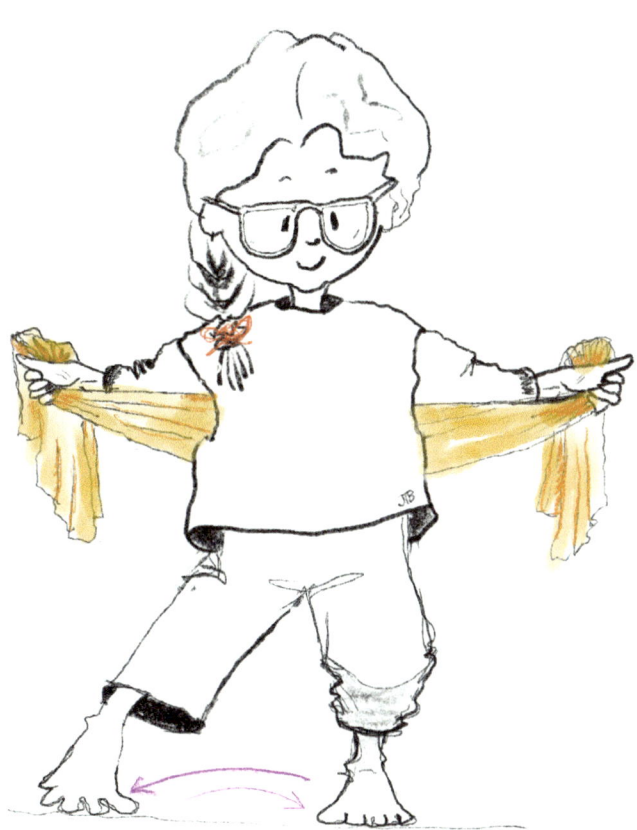

Figure 64 Recoil 3.4.

▶ *Variation 3:* The final progression of this sequence is to incorporate the spiralling figure-eight movement of the arms with the rebounding movement of the legs. Once there is competency in all the above, start by taking the right leg out to the side first, so the left arm will be making the figure-eight pattern. Notice that with the stride to the right and bringing the left arm across, the tension of the band increases, creating a natural recoiling that will spring and restore back to vertical and centre.

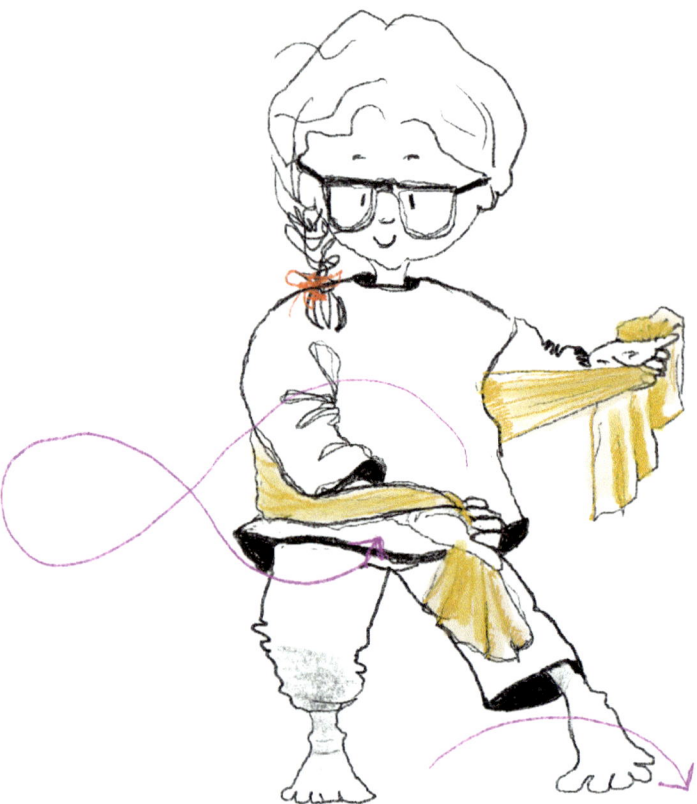

Figure 65 Recoil 3.5.

▶ *Variation 4:* Aim to be light on the feet and springy while recoiling under the natural tensional matrix that's been created. Finally, alternate between striding to the left and striding to the right.

PRACTICE SECTION 3: RELEASE

Release 1: self-regulation – subtle spine-tuning and why appropriate yawning counts

Purpose: Pandiculation as a means to influence myofascial release.

Support: If available, use a bolster or firm cushion, or sit on a chair. The key is not to collapse into the sitting position, but to feel supported from the ground up beyond the crown.

Timing: Work at a speed in which it is possible to track the sensations and any changes to the *texture* and *consistency* of the myofascial matrix and the inner sense of the responsiveness.

Sequence:

▸ Find a comfortable seated position (see support). Feel lengthened and supported through the spine.

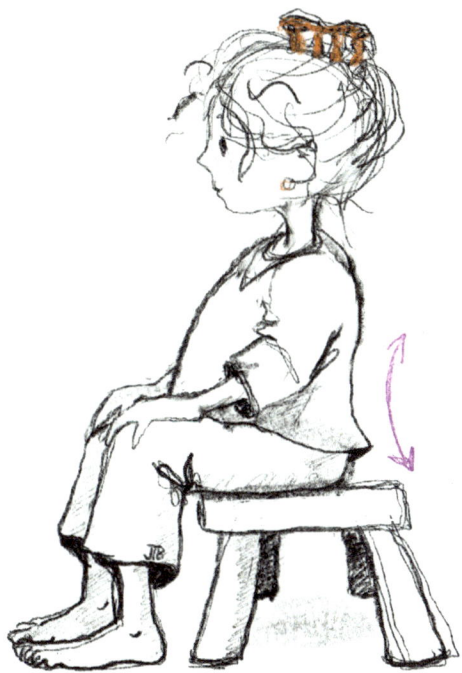

Figure 66 Release 1.1.

▸ Begin to roll the pelvis forwards and backwards, rocking over the sitting bones, noticing the natural response of the body, allowing room for the visceral tissues to move with the undulating motion of the pelvis. Breathe easily.

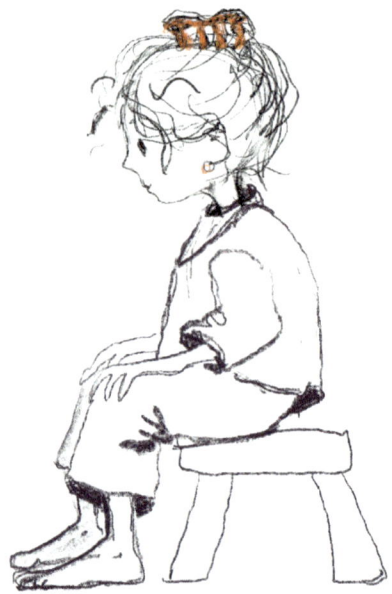

Figure 67 Release 1.2.

▸ Explore draping the torso forward over the legs, letting the arms hang toward the ground. Notice which way the pelvis has to move to accommodate this. (Does it tilt forwards or backwards?)

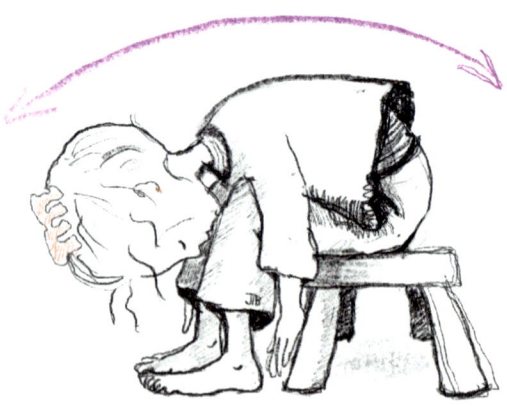

Figure 68 Release 1.3.

▸ Circle the whole torso over the base, in a clockwise and then counterclockwise direction. Notice any reflexive sensations in the torso
as the body circles and rotates sensing any restrictions. Feel into the
movements, without forcefulness, exploring if every direction is easy
or not. Work lightly so there is a deeper sense of any areas that feel
achy or sticky. This is not a twist in the torso, this is a stirring motion.
Imagine looking down onto the crown: the head and torso would be
drawing a circle shape around the pelvis, so the weight shifts from
side to front to side to back and then returning back the way it came.

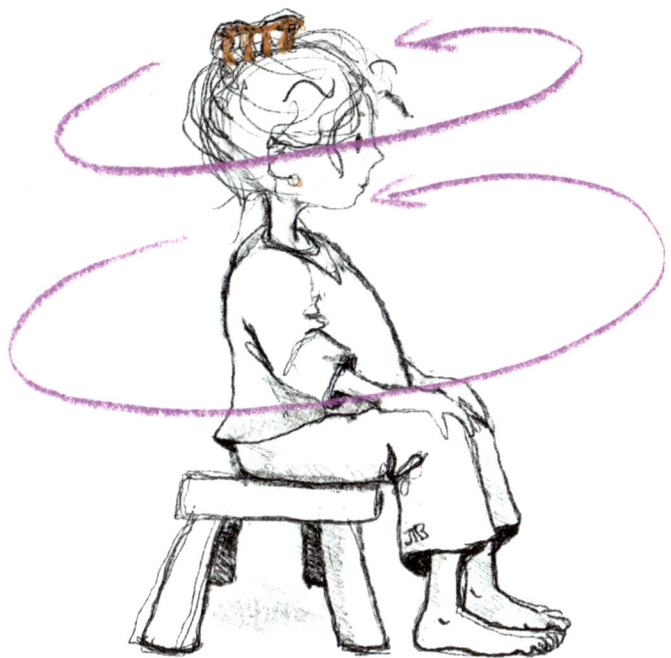

Figure 69 Release 1.4.

▸ Once the circling (circumduction) is explored in both directions, return to the centre. Here we begin to explore pandiculation – a yawning stretch. The actual 'yawn' is an essential part of the movement and can be added to any movements, standing, sitting, and lying down.

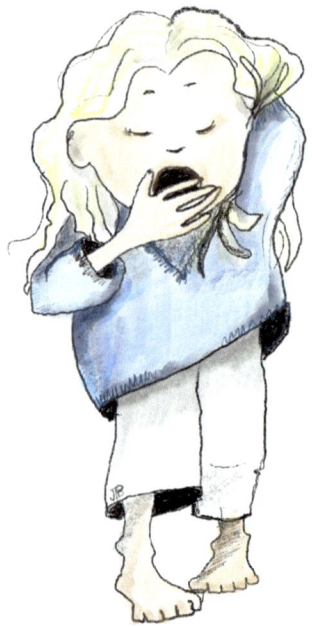

Figure 70 Release 1.5.

▸ Open the mouth wide, as if in a yawn, reaching and lengthening the arms away into the boundary of natural reach (no need to push beyond natural constraint or 'fasciategral limit'). Then bring the hands and arms together (while outstretched) and bend at the elbows to bring the hands towards the mouth. As the hands get closer together in front of the open mouth, sense the compression in the shoulders as they squeeze. This in turn will invite the yawn, which stimulates reaching away of the arms, outwardly in a big yawning gesture of unfolding. (This is somasensing through deep deceleration of the tissues.) Essentially, there is a feeling of 'reach and resist' (at the same time) which is the hallmark of myofascial deceleration. It is an exaggerated yawn. You can continue this in the sitting position. Add the legs and then move arms and legs together as you explore this. (This sequence animates the pandiculation/yawning effect.)

▸ It can be delightful to really explore this movement, making different shapes and allowing the body to move as it wants to. Perhaps it chooses to twist or curl, or push, or fold following the initiation of the mouth opening and widening. (This can of course be done lying supine and is a wonderful practice for a minute or two upon waking up, while in bed.)

▸ If the body feels like it cannot arch back, or reach in a particular direction, allow it to go where it can and does prefer. For example: if the body is predisposed to go (without resistance), into a forward fold (which is the most usual preference), then go towards that preference, even more deeply than might first seem enough. In other words, yawn into the preference. As this feeling deepens, it may be possible to come out of the yawn and reach gradually in the opposite direction more easily once you have deepened the yawning into the place the body prefers. This is a guided technique that can be adapted to 'feeling into how it feels more' – as if 'giving in' to the preferred way allows the body to feel reassured and heard. Coming out (without force and with gentle curiosity) can take the body to a place of relaxation and gradually it may feel rewarding to yawn and reach into an arch of extension more easily. Essentially, if someone is stuck in flexion, then taking that deeper in this considered way animates a new boundary to explore. In turn, this can become a new and more upright position. These mini sequences take time and patience; however, it is a very reassuring way for the body to explore relaxation, which serves the myofascial system enormously. (See Part 4: Release by John Sharkey.) This practice is not about finding range or reach. It is based in honouring the inner senses and preferences and exploring them, forgiving them, giving them the attention to go deeper. It is not about calling them to 'improve' or 'go further'. It is a completely 'person centred' and individual exercise (with many rewards if it is practised)! It can become a disproportionately valuable asset to all the other systems because it can, over time, release old postural habits born of default patterns associated with emotional defences as well as physical insults. The essential ingredient is to go with the body's preference, not against it, at all. It is not in competition with itself; it is seeking peace.

Release 2: supine curl – why slow counts

Purpose: Harnessing possible symmetries and asymmetries to support myofascial release.

Support: Use cushions, two bolsters, or a long rolled up blanket as supportive props.

Timing: Go slow to give the tissue the time to respond to the intentions. Encourage awareness of subtlety and nuance within the movement(s). There is nothing to achieve here, just listening.

Sequence:

▸ Using cushions, two bolsters, or a long rolled up blanket, (have the client) lie semi-supine (crown to tailbone) over their supportive prop, with their knees bent, feet standing (hip-width apart approximately) on the ground, and arms rested down by the sides.

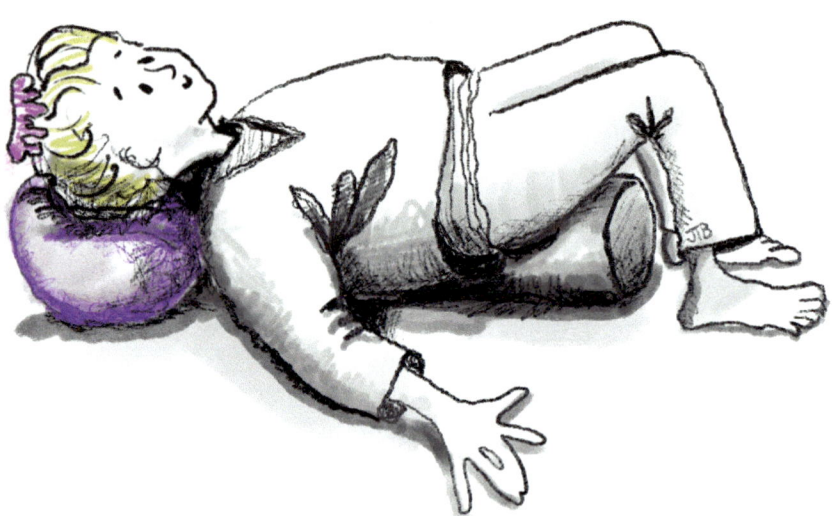

Figure 71 Release 2.1.

▸ Explore tilting the pelvis gently forwards and backwards, noticing any corresponding sensations in the neck (cervical spine) and head. Sense if there is a direct influence over subtle movement at the neck by initiating movement from the pelvis.

▸ Choosing either arm to begin, invite the arm upwards and backwards towards the floor behind the client. Move it backwards and forwards in a steady rhythm, finding a flow of motion. Play with the reach of the arm, direction of the fingertips, and the positioning of the palm of the hand to access the rotational spiralling network within, that allows the area being worked with to find natural myofascial release, or identify any restrictions. Work gently, without force and with curiosity. This movement is effectively winding and unwinding the natural rotation of the arms and the rhythm of the shoulder complex. Work to both sides.

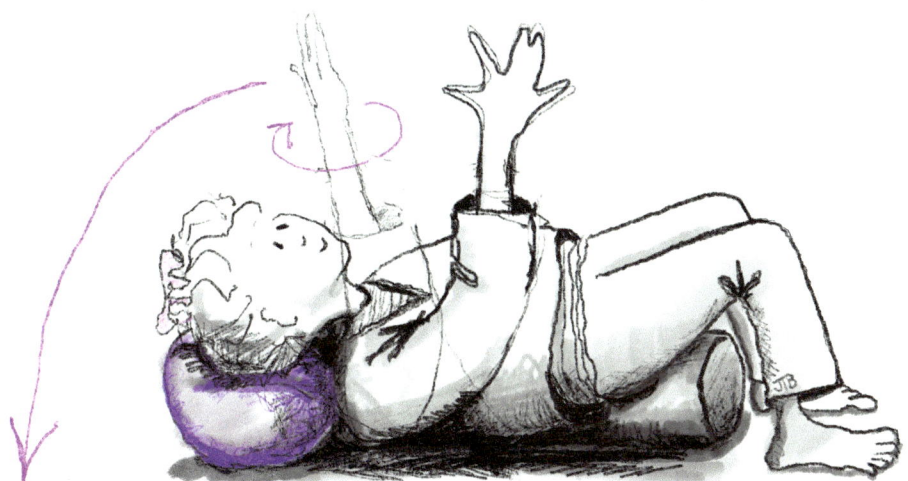

Figure 72 Release 2.2.

▸ *Variation 1:* The next step is to move both arms in opposition to each other, backwards and forwards whilst exploring rotation of the wrists, elbows and shoulders. If one arm is going up and over the head, then the other is going forward and down by the side. The arms are both twisting and recoiling through their length, while they alternate rotational direction from one to the other.

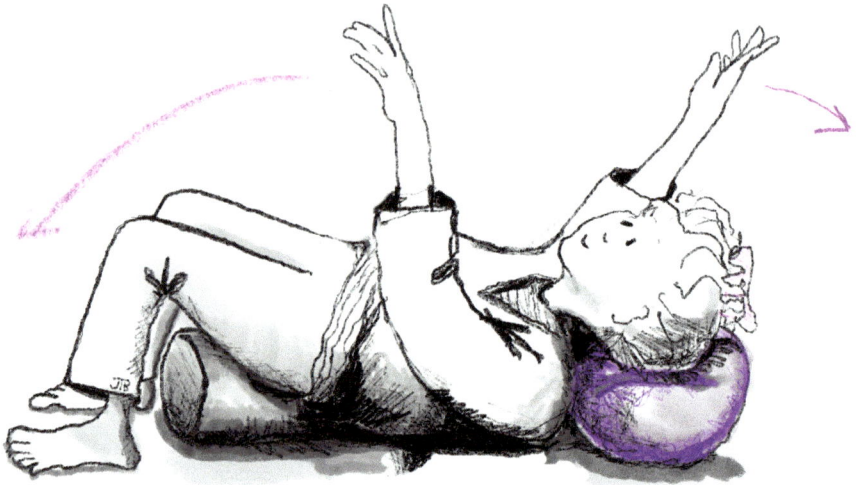

Figure 73 Release 2.3.

▸ *Variation 2:* Now try synchronizing the circling of the arms, bringing them both up in front of the supine torso, so the hands are pointing towards the ceiling, back behind the head and down along the sides of the body. Loop the movements in variations of figures-of-eight (out to the sides and across the torso).

▸ *Variation 3:* Is it possible to explore different textures through the arms, along a spectrum of softness to stiffness while moving them through space? Recognize what maintains calm self-regulation and move at a pace where the sensations can be tracked and followed, noticing subtle changes as they come and go. This is establishing biomotional intelligence, as the awareness tracks the sensations of keeping the arms stiff from fingers to shoulder and seeing what happens when they are soft and even soggy. It brings awareness of how there is an optimal way to feel in command of the movements, without restricting the arms or being too controlled about the movements. Let the arms provide information.

▸ *Variation 4:* The next progression of the arm movement is to continue circling the arms at the appropriate 'set' between stiffness and softness. This time move the arms in opposition to each other, creating a windmill effect.

▸ *Variation 5:* Bring the arms down to rest by the sides. Place the feet sole-to-sole. Now bring attention to the legs, let the knees come together, and then take them wide apart, in a rotational expression. Avoid allowing the knees to 'collapse' into the movement in either direction. This can be done one leg at a time, or both together, listening to the changes.

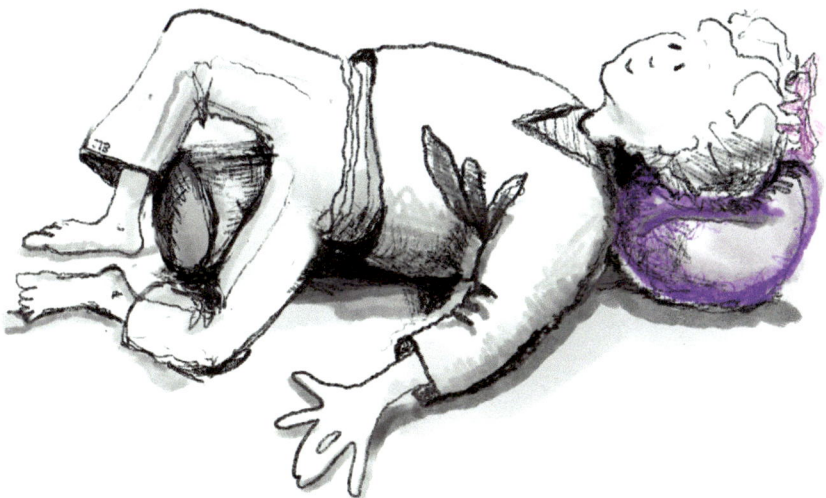

Figure 74 Release 2.4.

▸ *Variation 6:* Now bring one foot off the ground and fold at the knee, bringing it towards the chest with the hands interlaced around the back of the thigh (behind the knee) for support. Feel into the effect along the spine on that side. Take a little time to feel into it. Place that foot back on the floor and then repeat on the other side.

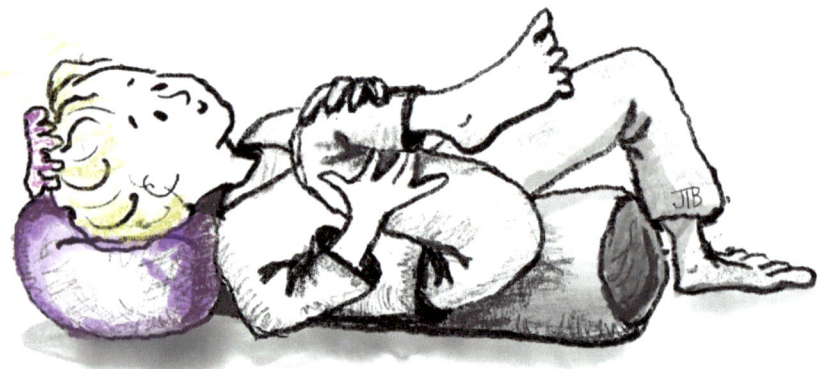

Figure 75 Release 2.5.

▸ After experiencing both sides, bring both legs in towards the chest, with the hands around the knees or behind them around the thighs for comfort. The knees can be together or wide, whatever is most comfortable for the individual. Rest in this position for a moment or two, ensuring comfort and balance on the props being used.

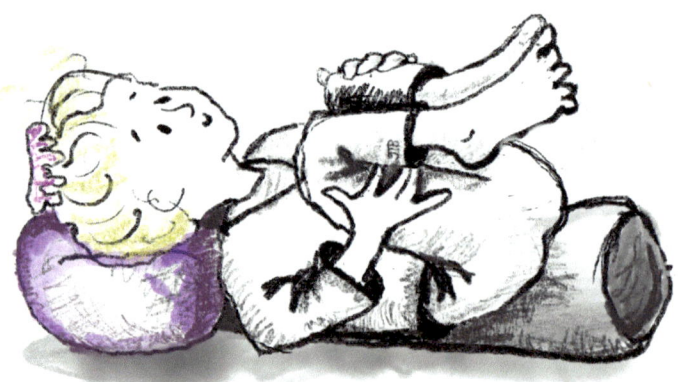

Figure 76 Release 2.6.

▸ *Practitioner note: If the client is not experienced in using bolsters, it is advisable to use flatter cushions or a towel or blanket under the body.*

▸ *Variation 7:* This variation brings the body into a forward folded curl (flexion). Slowly bring the chest and eyeline towards the navel, allowing the breath to have an internal influence as the client pauses in this curled position. Feel the expansion on the in-breathe and open into the foundation beneath the torso. Notice on the out-breath if it is possible to deepen into the curl.

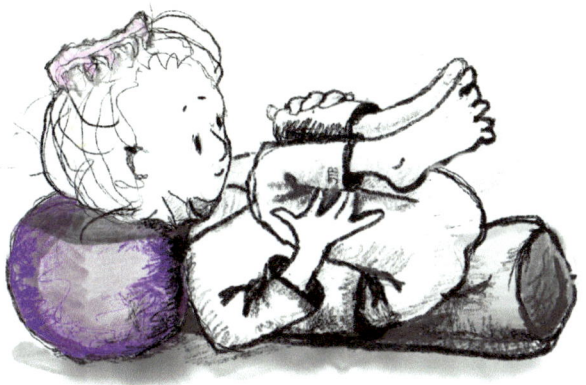

Figure 77 Release 2.7.

▸ To come out of this position, bring the head back to the bolster, then place one foot down at a time before uncurling the thoracic spine back to rest fully on the supportive prop.

▸ Rest and assess before rolling to one side to sit up, using the hands to rise.

Release 3: four-point kneeling – why rotation counts

Purpose: Playful motion to explore restrictions within movement, gently utilizing forces – both external and internal – to communicate with the tissues, inviting space, folding, yield, tensioning, and rotation. These are super valuable somasensing practices.

Support: Active contact through the ground print is offering support through the whole structure. Make sure there is a comfortable surface to work on, using extra padding if necessary.

Timing: Exploratory, finding a rhythm to the forwards and backwards motion, unique to the person practising.

Sequence:

▸ Position on all fours with the hands slightly forward of the shoulders, knees comfortably under the hips and toes tucked under (if comfortable) with the heels pointing upward.

▸ Explore the sensation of pushing through the hands to round the upper spine, and then the opposite movement, which is dropping the spine between the shoulders as the back arches. With sensitivity to the touch, push through the hands until it is easy to organize the thoracic spine between the shoulders, where it is neither over tensioned (rounded) nor collapsed (arched). *This is a refined balance, a point between extremes, that requires focus until it becomes natural.* It is sometimes referred to as a 'neutral spine', however, it is less of a position than a feeling from the inside of somasensing readiness or poise with the freedom to move equally smoothly into both an arch or a curl from that place.

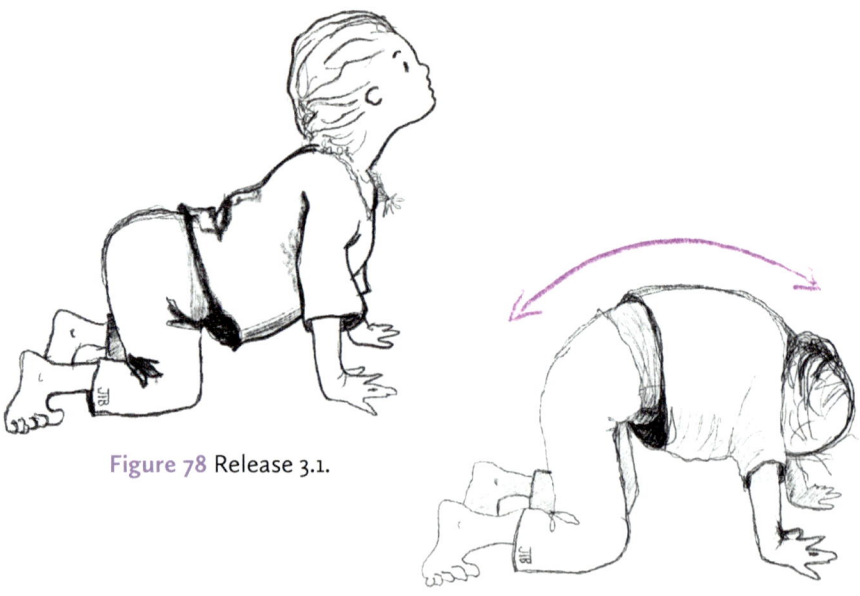

Figure 78 Release 3.1.

Figure 79 Release 3.2.

▶ Imagine the spine is growing out beyond the crown of the head and the tail, creating appropriate tensional balance to animate the tissues along the full length of the back body (feeling as if the *somasense* of the spine goes beyond the head and tail). Make sure the head is aligned with the cervical spine. (Not arched or rounded at the neck.)

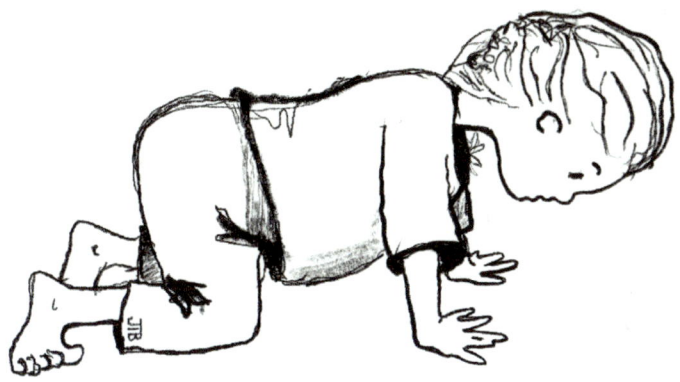

Figure 80 Release 3.3.

▶ Start to sway the body from side to side (shifting the weight from right knee/hand to left knee/hand), noticing how the push and pull of the outer hands facilitate the movement of rocking.

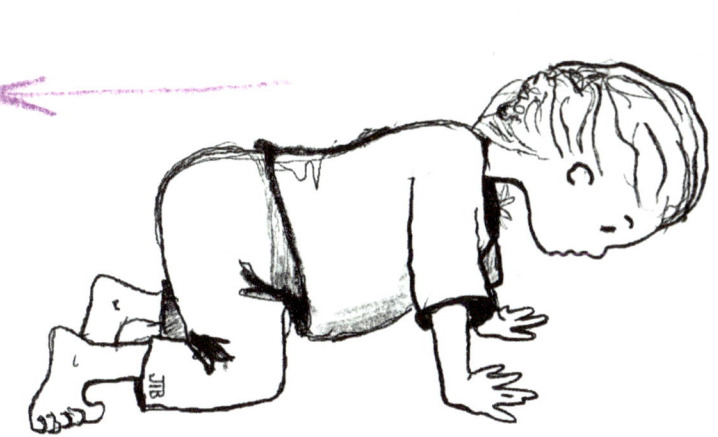

Figure 81 Release 3.4.

▶ *Variation 1:* follow the side-to-side rocking by creating circular movements in a clockwise direction over the entire ground print. This will
be a gentle moving forwards and backwards, as well as side to side.
Make sure that the spine does not collapse but invite it to respond to
the shifting of the weight. Somasense is being deepened and micro-
tuned here. Repeat in the other direction (counterclockwise).

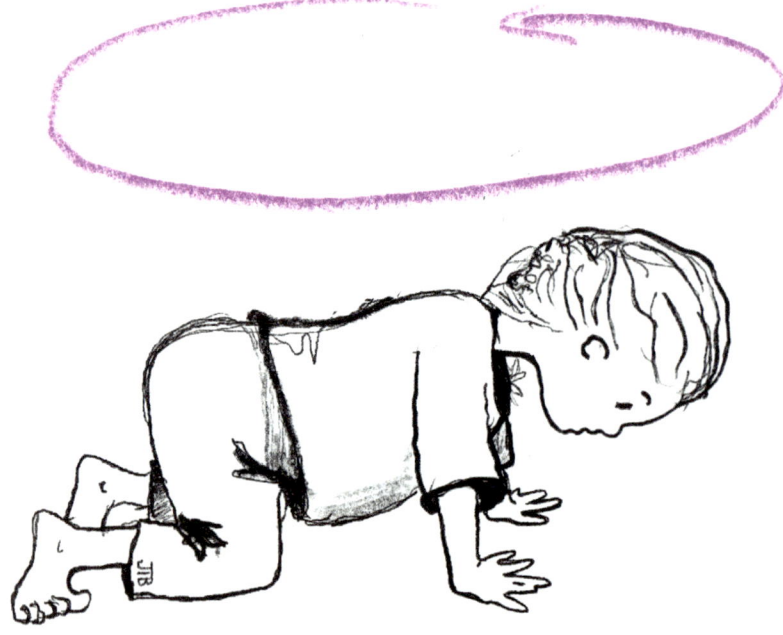

Figure 82 Release 3.5.

▶ *Variation 2:* Return to centre, and now take the weight forwards and
backwards, over the hands and back towards the heels. Once there
is an established rhythm, explore taking one hand off the ground,
swinging it back behind while shifting the weight towards the heel.
At the same time, allow the spine to round, followed by swinging
the arm forward and lengthening it in front to bring the weight over
the hands.

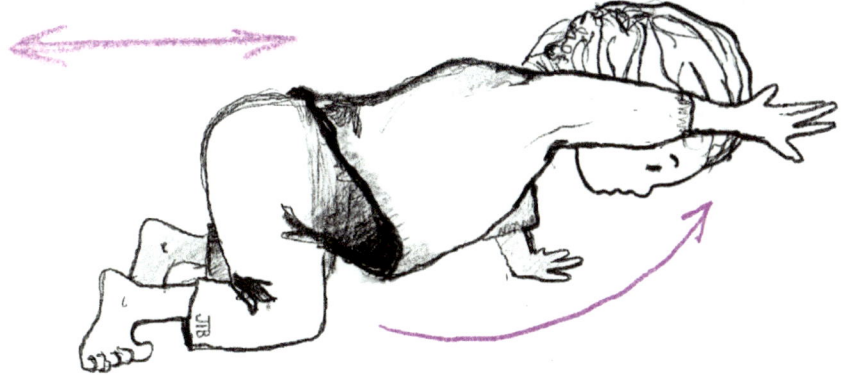

Figure 83 Release 3.6.

▶ *Variation 3:* Return to the neutral position. Bring one hand across the body to touch the *opposite* knee, resting the elbow of that (same) arm on the *same side* knee. (It will be necessary to fold at the knees, slightly more deeply, and take the weight back towards the heels to accommodate this movement.) Release the arm and lengthen it in front to pull the weight back over the standing hand. Now repeat this sequence, establishing a rhythm to the movement. Notice that the *underlying* micro-pattern is the shifting of the weight forward and backwards, challenged slightly by the arm reaching forward and folding back in a diagonal crossbody motion. Repeat on the other side.

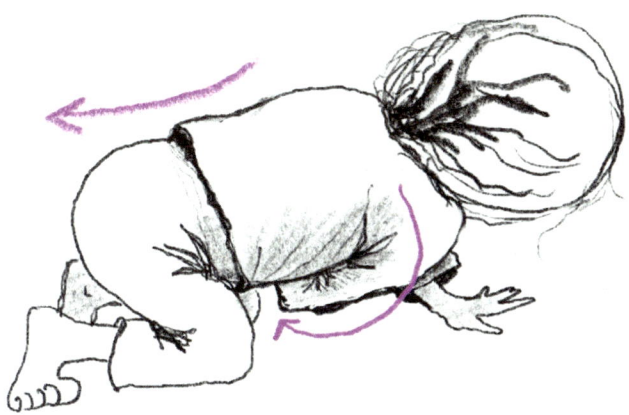

Figure 84 Release 3.7.

▸ *Variation 4:* The next progression is to bring the *elbow* (rather than the hand) to the opposite knee while shifting the weight backwards, then lengthening the arm fully out in front of the ground print, to bring the weight back over the standing hand. Once again, find a rhythm to this playful movement. Don't force it and if it is too much for a participant, simply stay at Variation 3. To support deeper rotation of the thoracic body, try not to shift the weight to one side, staying present to the geometry of the support shape being made, including the ground print. Repeat on the other side. (This is a deep subtle move *towards* the possibility of reaching the elbow to opposite knee. It is not to be forced.)

▸ Make sure that the ribs are not rolling or bending off to the side to find this crossbody motion. We do not want to sacrifice clarity for achievement. Organize the ribs centrally to optimize their rotation. It is better to work gently towards this possibility than 'achieve' it, by going beyond fasciategral range and overreaching. Explore breathing into the shape being made here and possibly bringing the weight further back, if that is comfortable. Be careful not to collapse, but maintain the integrity of the fasciategral forces being transmitted through the whole body.

Release 4: reciprocal release

Purpose: Exploring myofascial release through side-bending, flexion, and extension patterns.

Support: Stability ball.

Timing: Explorative. Repeat the sequences as appropriate, doing them to both sides. This is not a stretching exercise but an invitation for the tissues to respond appropriately, exploring the sense of structural integrity while creating the conditions to prevent stiffening or collapsing.

Sequence:

▸ Place a stability ball onto the outside of the hip, pressing into it with the wrist. This will help maintain integrity within the myofascial architecture, whilst giving 'feedback in space' of where the position is and what direction to move into. (It is somasensing feedback.)

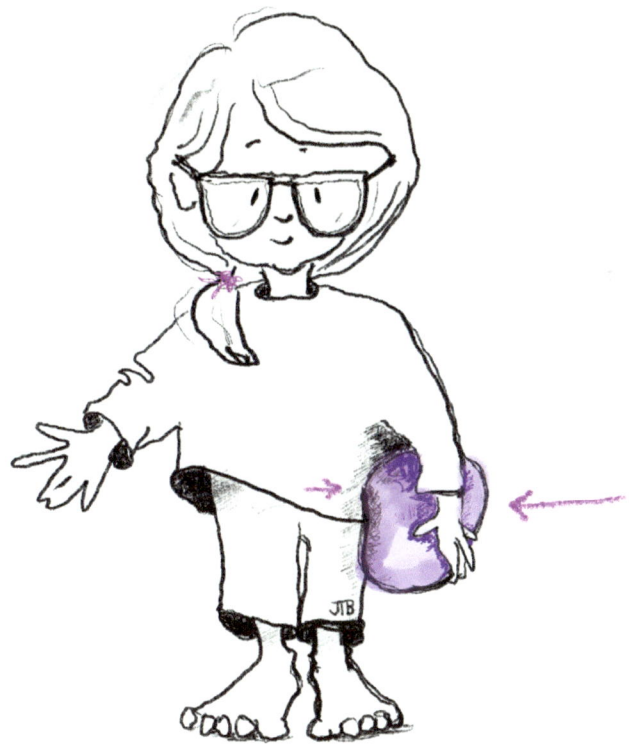

Figure 85 Release 4.1.

▸ Make sure that the hip is reciprocally pressing back; sense equal pressure from the outer thigh towards the wrist, as the wrist towards the outer thigh, through the ball.

▸ Reach and lengthen the free arm into the air above the head, cultivating a sense of tensegral reaction upward, to the compressive force of gravity that is working in a downwards direction. Don't 'stretch', rather find the fasciategral range that feels 'just' right.

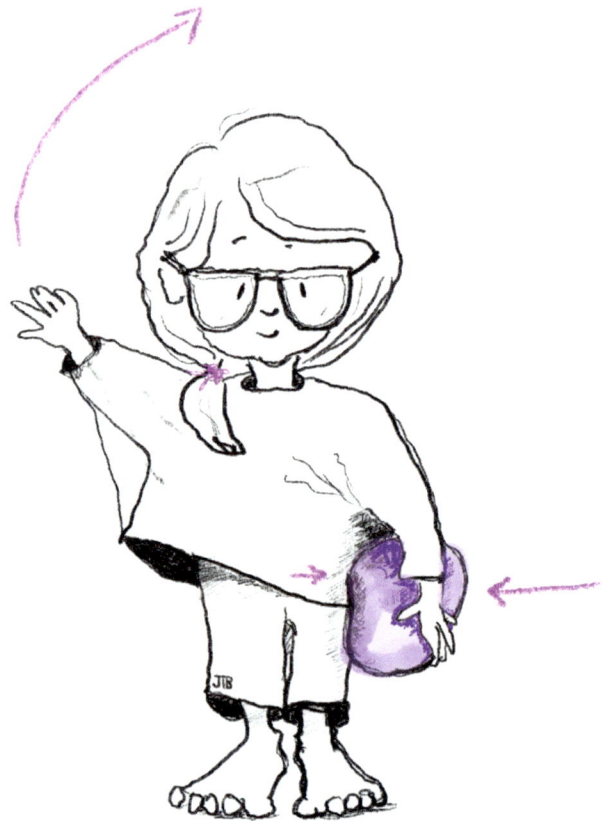

Figure 86 Release 4.2.

▸ *Variation 1:* Maintain the reach through the up-reached arm whilst softening the shoulder and begin tilting the head away from that arm, towards the same side that the ball is placed. There is a somasense of the neck *lengthening in that direction*, not folding or collapsing. Now gradually follow that direction with the ribs and free arm whilst continuing to press the pelvis into the ball (simultaneously the ball presses into the side of the pelvis; it needs to feel like a mutually compressive balance between the hip and the wrist). This balance with the ball helps to maintain integrity of the tubular torso. Do not 'drop' or 'collapse' into that side or send the hip sideways. The pelvic girdle (hips) stays above the feet, resisting the ball and 'pushing back' into the wrist, just enough to maintain structural integrity of the whole frame.

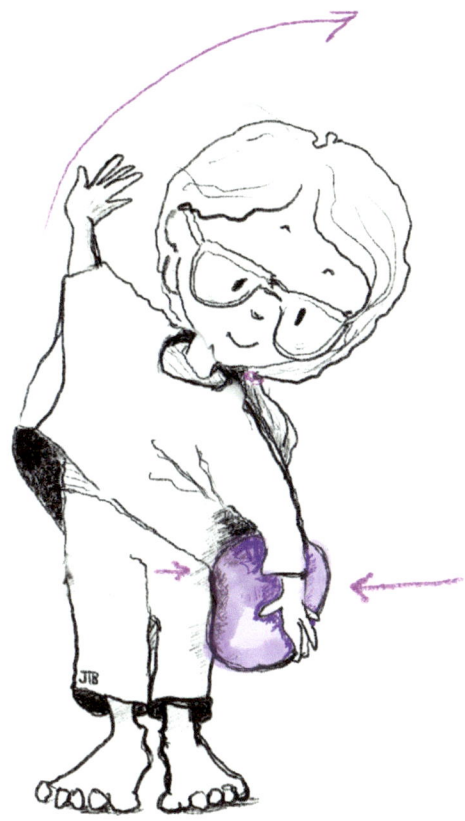

Figure 87 Release 4.3.

▸ To return to standing, lengthen up through the thoracic and then the cervical spine, bringing the body back to neutral with the free arm maintained in a vertical position. Then lower it, so the client is going back the way they came. Repeat the movement to continue the exploration of myofascial release, a few times without strain. Let the arm rest by the side and release the ball, sensing the shape of that side of the body, from ground to crown. (Pause to do this before doing the other side – it helps to appreciate the difference!)

▸ Repeat this sequence on the other side.

This effectively releases suboptimal postural patterns between the pelvic and shoulder girdles in relation to the ground. Without overtly 'thinking' through the posture, it animates the side body to optimize tubular balance through somasense of the whole torso and ground-to-crown organization. The point is not necessarily to overtly direct the body (verbally) but to build the subtle experience through movement practice, to optimize integrity throughout the form.

Release 5: positional release (stillness)
This can be used at any point in any class where rest is optimal between sequences or after completion. It is designed to promote full recovery for body, breath, and being.

Purpose: Passive positional myofascial release.

Support: Stability ball, cushions, or two bolsters.

Timing: This is a great opportunity to become quiet and find stillness, whilst staying aware of any subtle shifts to the physiology through taking the time to actively rest. Stay in this position for as long as feels comfortable or according to how much time is available.

Sequence:

▸ In side-lying position, place a stability ball or cushion underneath the head (deflated enough that the neck is not side-bent when resting the head on the ball), cushions or a bolster underneath the top bent leg, and cushions or a bolster underneath the top bent arm. Make sure the rest of the body feels comfortable (use a towel, cushions, or blanket if optimal).

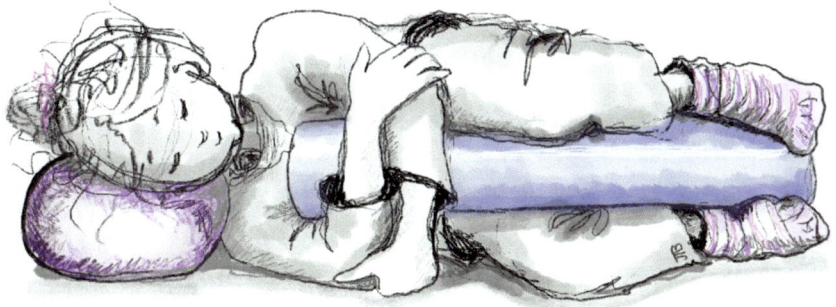

Figure 88 Release 5.1.

▸ Feeling fully supported by the props and the ground beneath the whole body, observe the quality of the breath and how the myofascial matrix responds to the organization of the body, with nothing else to do besides noticing. There is nothing to do here. Simply be. It is bonus time for the body.

PRACTICE SECTION 4: RESTORE

Restore 1: restoring vertical

Purpose: Integrating verticality and myofascial integrity through the torso to support breath, structure, and visceral organs in everyday posture.

Support: Chair and/or stability ball.

Timing: Take the time to explore the sensations, enjoying the attentive, compassionate quality of restoring true vertical alignment to the tissue matrix, especially for sitting poses that are required to travel or work at a desk.

Sequence:

▸ Sit on a firm chair either in the middle or towards the front of the seat, so that the feet can rest directly underneath the knees. Place the hands on the thighs and apply a downward push through the feet and the hands to create a vertical counter-response through the spine. Practise releasing the pressure and seeing how the body responds, then repeat the movement, continuing to loop the actions (pressing and releasing) while finding a rhythm. The push gesture is not aggressive, it is sensitive, and the purpose is to explore the sensations of *somasense feedback*. This is a finessing technique that builds subtle awareness and control so that the body can respond more optimally when there is variability of motion.

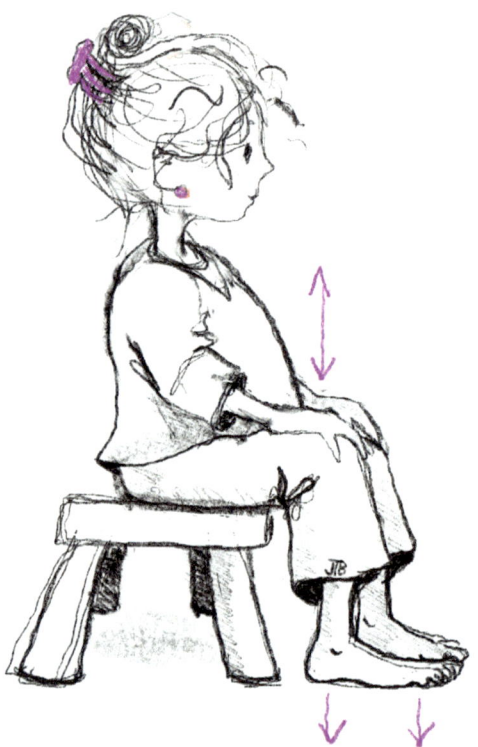

Figure 89 Restore 1.1.

▶ *Variation 1:* Add the breath awareness. Explore these actions with the breath, inhaling as the hands press downwards through to the feet, rising naturally. Then exhale to descend equally thoughtfully, without collapsing back onto the chair or ball. Stay attentive to the rhythm.

▸ *Variation 2:* Taking the stability ball and holding it lightly against the body with flat hands in the lap, roll the ball upwards gently pressing against the abdomen with the inhale so it mimics the rising of the rib cage, then roll it back down to the lap with the exhale, as the ribs descend.

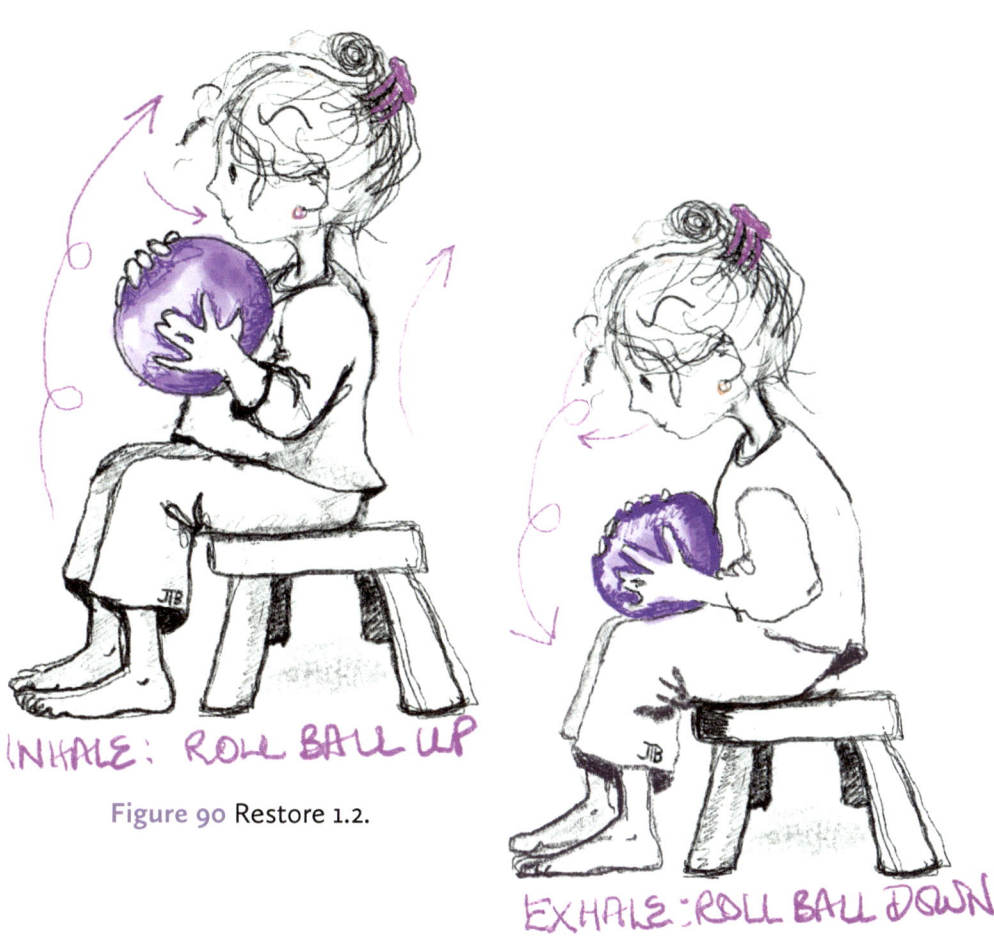

INHALE: ROLL BALL UP

Figure 90 Restore 1.2.

EXHALE: ROLL BALL DOWN

Figure 91 Restore 1.3.

Restore 2: restoring rotation

Purpose: Restoring awareness of rotational bias and optimizing natural and appropriate inhibition.

Support: Use a bolster if needed to support the verticality, otherwise you can sit on a chair or on the floor with the legs comfortably crossed.

Timing: Over the course of the exploration, notice if qualities of ease and glide are restored to the rotational movement.

Sequence:

▸ In the chosen seated position, cross the hands over, either resting them on the chest or folding the forearms on top of each other like a genie, or placing them on the belly. The purpose is to activate the arms to feel into the continuity of the shoulders and thorax.

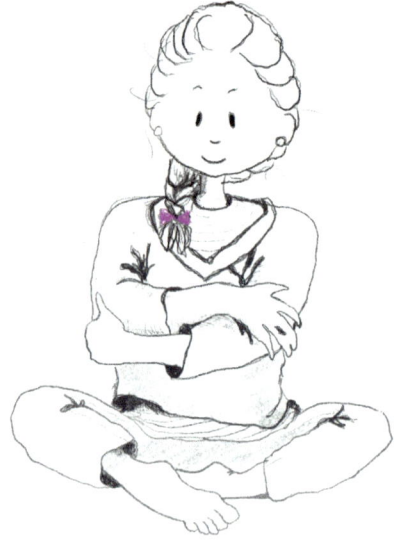

Figure 92 Restore 2.1.

▸ Begin to rotate gently towards the right, then towards the left, noticing the natural barrier (the point of resistance) that the body is creating according to the arrangement of the legs. (This changes with different leg positions, which is explored here.)

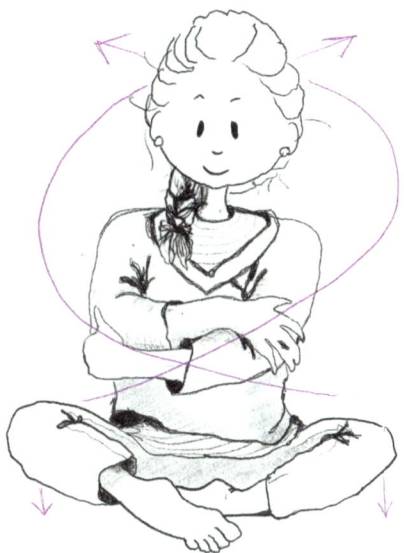

Figure 93 Restore 2.2.

▸ Now cross the legs the other way around (whichever one was underneath is now on top) and, swapping the arms, repeat the same rotational exploration again, rotating the torso and arms. Notice restrictions and sensations of ease. Which direction are they?

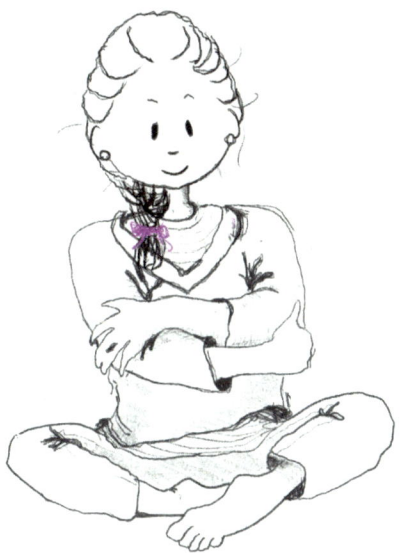

Figure 94 Restore 2.3.

▸ *Variation 1:* Either keeping the legs as they are or swapping the legs over again, let the breath now accompany the movement. As the rotation begins, inhale through the nose, and exhale through the mouth as the rotation comes back to the centre. Practise this from side to side, working with the breath in a qualitative way to support expansion of the ribs while rotating. Notice a possible feeling of release when encouraging a slightly longer exhale.

▸ Repeat this sequence again, changing the legs this time (and the arms, as above). It is important to keep the legs awake. The legs must be active in their downward contact with the ground to maintain the counterbalance, which animates verticality through the torso.

▸ *Practitioner note: If working with a client, ask their permission to place your hands underneath the sides of the ribs by kneeling behind them, to offer a gentle upwards lift so the ribs feel as though they are growing up and out of the pelvis, using the hands to gently guide their rotation, without forcing at all, beyond the natural constraint. This is not about overcoming constraint; rather it is focused on understanding, respecting, and honouring it to work within it and grow confidence.*

Restore 3: restore with the ball and the wall

Purpose: Restorative positioning of head, thorax, and pelvis to support walking and general movement.

Support: Wall, stability ball.

Timing: Explore each element of this sequence with the intention that you are not only restoring myofascial–neurological patterns of movement, but also conscious awareness of bodily relationships and the sense of self in space through restoring spinal organization. Practise, while maintaining a quality of attention that is fully present and curious. This seems very simple; however, it can have a deep and helpful effect once mastered.

Sequence:

▶ Start by standing a few inches from the wall and placing the ball behind the head, against the wall. There should be enough distance between the back of the heels and the wall so that the ball is not pushing the head forward of the feet. Feet are approximately hip width apart. Notice how the feedback of the ball helps to improve awareness of the standing posture throughout the body.

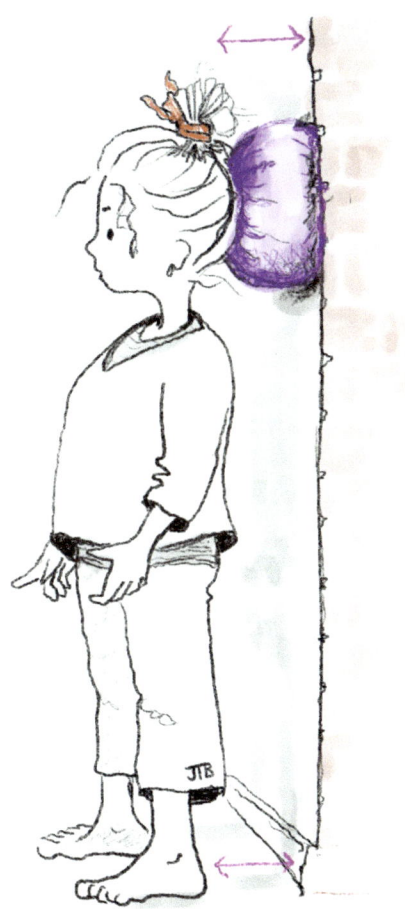

Figure 95 Restore 3.1.

▶ *Practitioner note: If working with a client, help position the ball for them, relative to the distance of the heels from the wall. It should be 'just right' so the ball is held between head and wall and the heels are under the back of the cranium.*

▶ Start to play with micro-movements of the head at the level of the occipital ridge, which is approximately in line with the ears. This is where motion of the skull on top of the spine occurs. Micro-move the head up and down, side to side, and rotate left and right. Let the head yield with the ball to accommodate the micro-movements. Begin to increase the range of motion with the head, without moving the rest of the body, while keeping the ball in place against the wall.

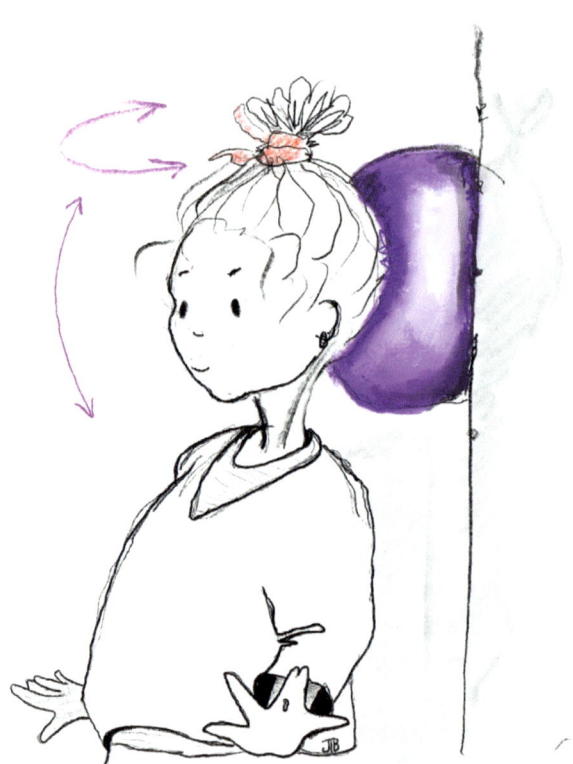

Figure 96 Restore 3.2.

▶ *Variation 1:* Keeping the head in contact with the ball against the wall, now lift the heel of one foot (leave the toes in contact with the floor), changing the proprioceptive feedback of the positioning in relationship with the ball. Alternate rhythmically, lifting one heel then the other.

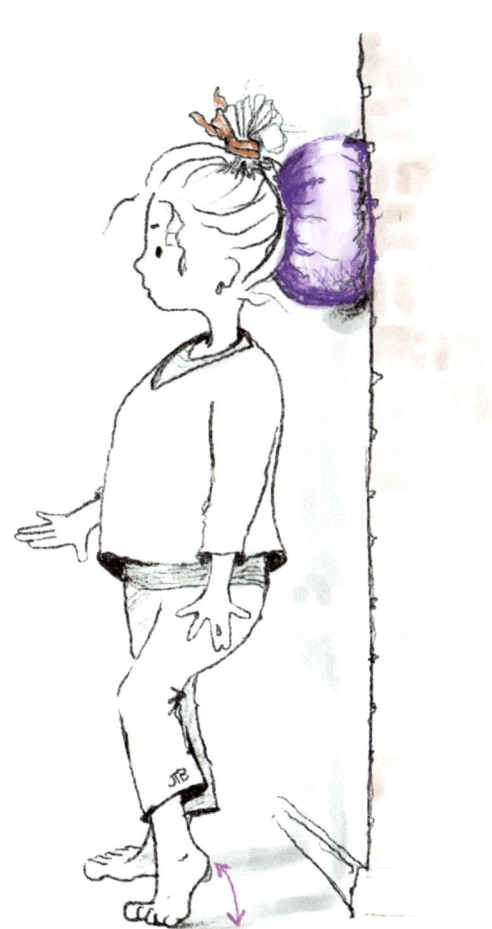

Figure 97 Restore 3.3.

▶ *Variation 2:* Place the feet close together, so they are just apart at the ankle. Make the same movement (lifting only the heel of each foot) with the feet together, raising one heel at a time. This helps to subtly re-educate and optimize the balance for contralateral walking.

▶ *Variation 3:* Maintaining a feet-together standing position, whilst still receiving the sensory feedback between the head and the ball, raise one heel off the ground feeling the weight shift to the other leg before raising the toes, too, so that the foot is entirely off the ground, bringing that leg up in front of the pelvis by bending the knee and lifting. Keep the movement streamlined and smooth, if possible.

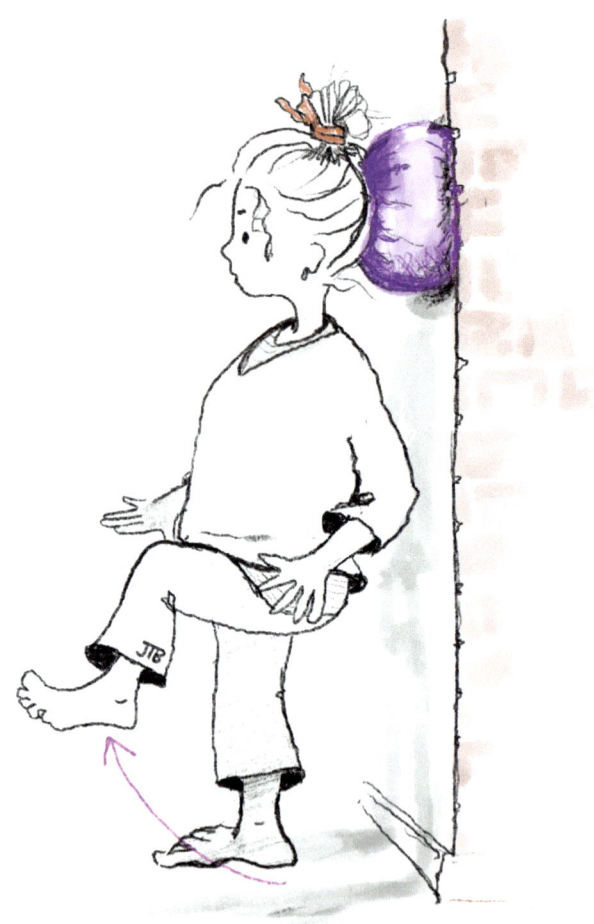

Figure 98 Restore 3.4.

▸ Maintaining weight through the standing leg, lightly return the foot back to the ground keeping the heel raised, toes spread wide before letting the heel gently return to the ground. Decelerate the movement as clearly and as precisely as doing (accelerating) it. Once both feet are on the ground, re-centre the weight so that it is evenly distributed through both legs. Repeat on the other side.

▸ *Variation 4:* Now move the ball to the middle thorax, approximately between the shoulder blades and behind the heart. With the arms in front of the body as though on a cross-trainer, start to explore rotation of the ribs from left to right 'around' the ball, while keeping it against the wall and holding the arms out in front of the body.

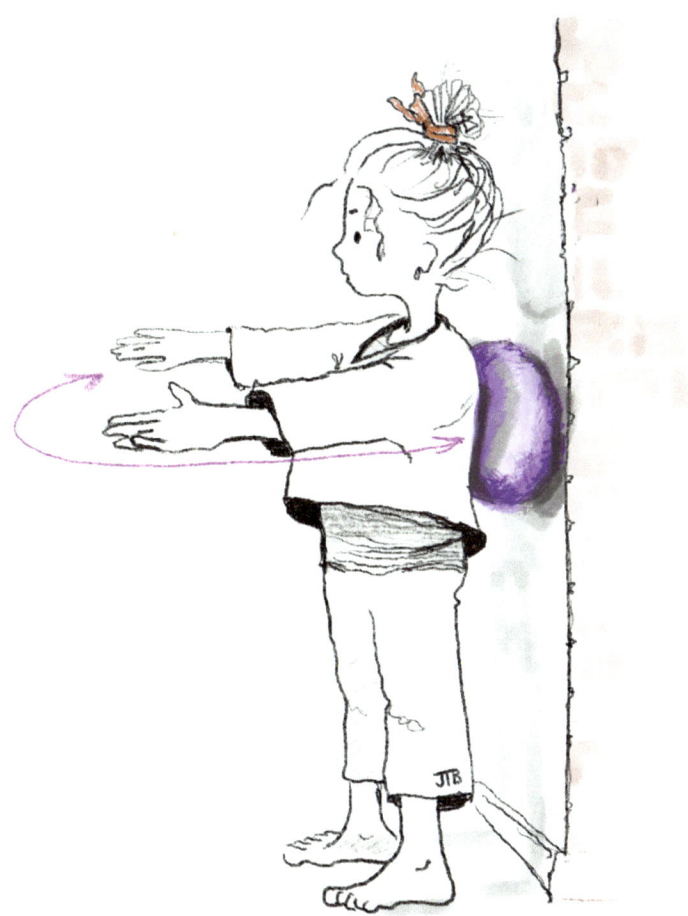

Figure 99 Restore 3.5.

▶ *Variation 5:* Invite the legs to join in, taking one heel up at a time as the arms swing and the thorax rotates (just the heels, one at a time, not the whole foot). *Whichever heel is off the ground, the opposite shoulder needs to be swinging forward to restore contralateral movement.* (This is essential.) Keep the ball against the wall behind the thoracic spine.

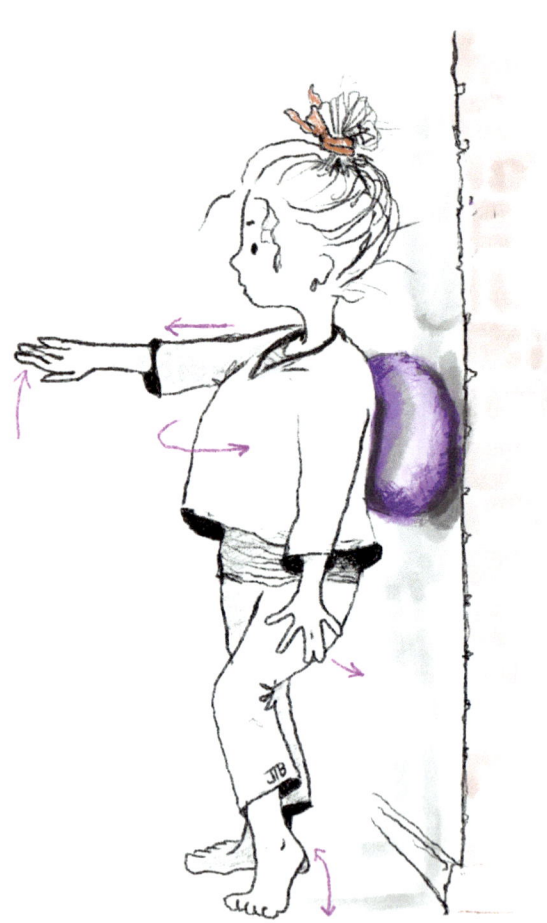

Figure 100 Restore 3.6.

▶ *Variation 6:* The next progression is to lift each foot entirely off the ground while 'walking' and maintaining contact and sensory awareness of the ball behind the thorax, holding it to the wall.

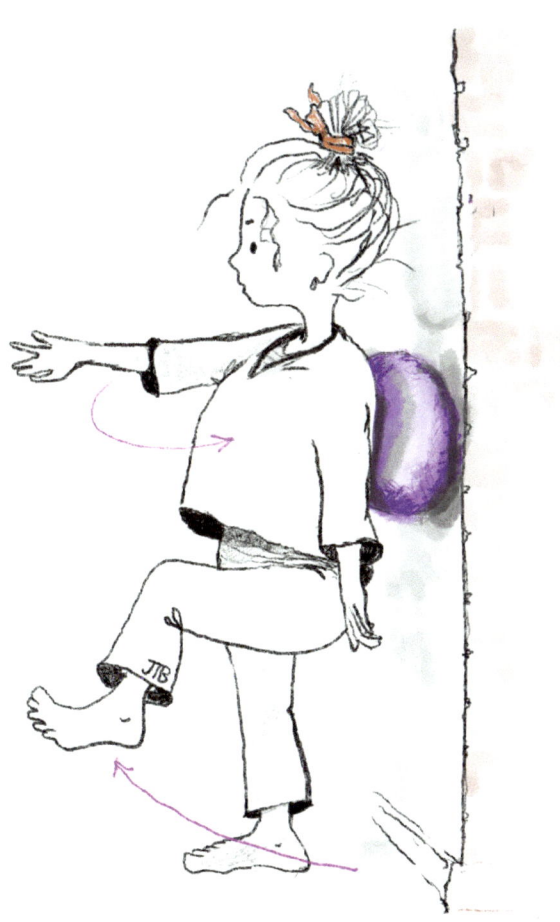

Figure 101 Restore 3.7.

▶ *Variation 7:* Now take the ball in the right hand and place it onto
the left thigh. As the left leg rises (bringing the foot off the ground),
use the ball to push the right hand forward and take the left arm
back, re-enforcing the rotation and contralateral pattern of the body.
Continue to lower and lift the leg in orchestration with the thorax
and arms, keeping the eye gaze facing forward to restore a deep sense
of counter rotational forces. Repeat on the other side (taking the ball
in the left hand and place it on the right thigh).

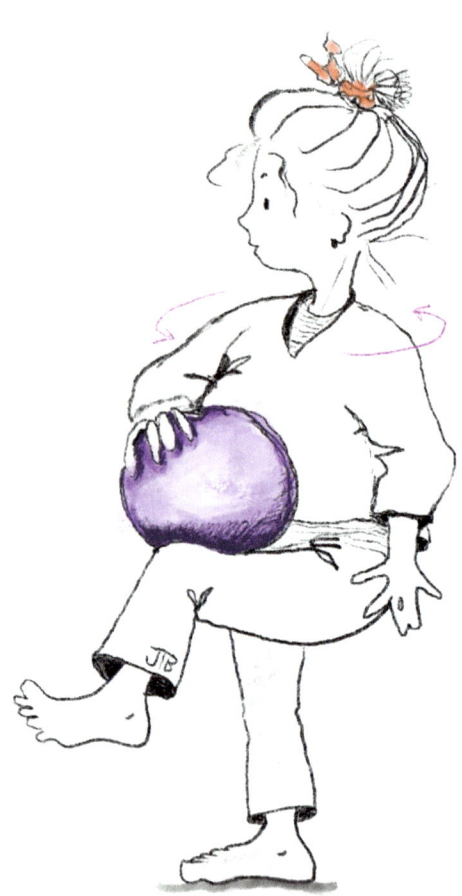

Figure 102 Restore 3.8.

▶ *Variation 8:* Place the ball behind the body, between the sacrum and the wall, keeping the body upright and just in front of the wall. Begin to rock the pelvis from side to side, transferring weight from one foot to the other. (Side-to-side lateral motion, not spiralling.)

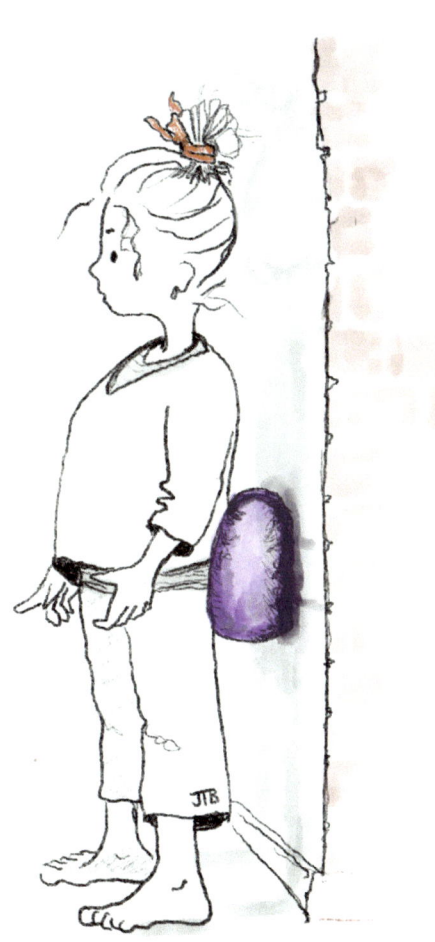

Figure 103 Restore 3.9.

▸ Return to neutral standing (with the ball between the sacrum and the wall) and begin to bend forward *without* pushing the ball into the wall. (This takes practise at first.) Notice what the pelvis *must do* to accommodate flexion of the spine without pushing the pelvis backwards. Unfurl the spine back up into standing. Repeat this a few times to give the body this foundational reminder of how to restore spinal integrity. (It looks simpler than it is at first.)

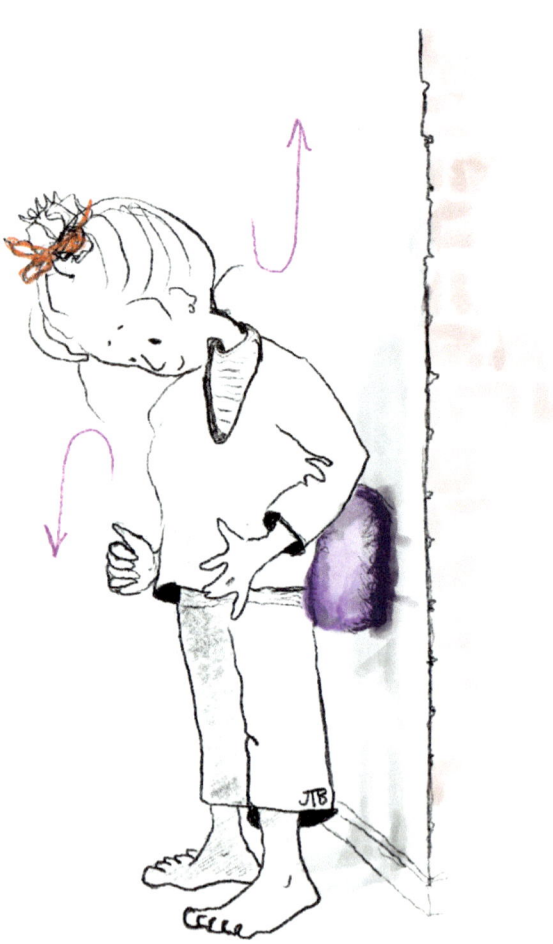

Figure 104 Restore 3.10.

Use this last exercise (especially after all the previous ones in this sequence) to explore articulation of the spine. It is *not* about reaching the hands to the toes! The flexion pattern is meant to be limited, perhaps more than might ordinarily be experienced in a movement class. The purpose of this is not to reach the floor or demonstrate the extent of forward bending. It is to bring articulation through the spine from crown to coccyx (head to tail), honouring the natural contralateral blueprint of human walking. It restores a lovely freedom of movement when incorporated into any practice.

PRACTICE SECTION 5: REFINE

Refine 1: refining forces through the arms via the ground

Purpose: Learning how to lower down with the arms.

Support: Using the ground.

Timing: Not counting reps but working self-regulating timeframes and body form. (Please note these are not press-ups!)

Sequence:

▶ Position on all fours, making sure the work is on a comfortable surface. Organize the hands slightly forward of the shoulders and be mindful of where the head is in relation to the upper spine; don't let the head hang. Make sure that there is no dropping in the lower spine, that the active contact being made through the ground print can offer subtle reorganization of the spine in this orientation. (Don't let the spine drop or arch between the shoulder blades – this is a position of somasensing integrity and balance.)

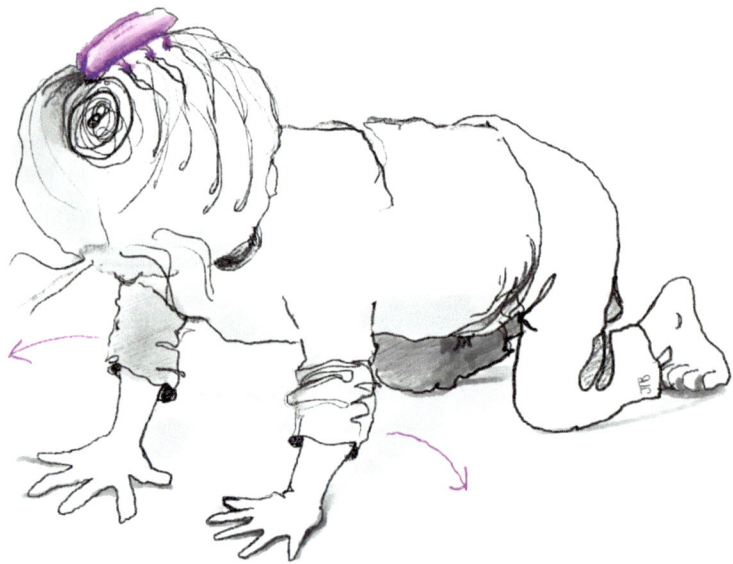

Figure 105 Refine 1.1.

▸ Once the all-fours position is refined, start to retract and protract the shoulders, bringing the shoulder blades inward (medial) towards the spine then away (lateral) from the spine, exploring the scapula range of motion, before resting with them in a central position, between retraction and protraction. There is a 'middle place' where they feel 'at home' – neither too close, nor too far from the spine. This is a small motion – it doesn't include the spine lifting or lowering, only the gliding of the shoulder blades.

▸ Next, bend the elbows whilst keeping the shoulder blades in their mid-position, without drawing them closer together. Repeat this movement a few times.

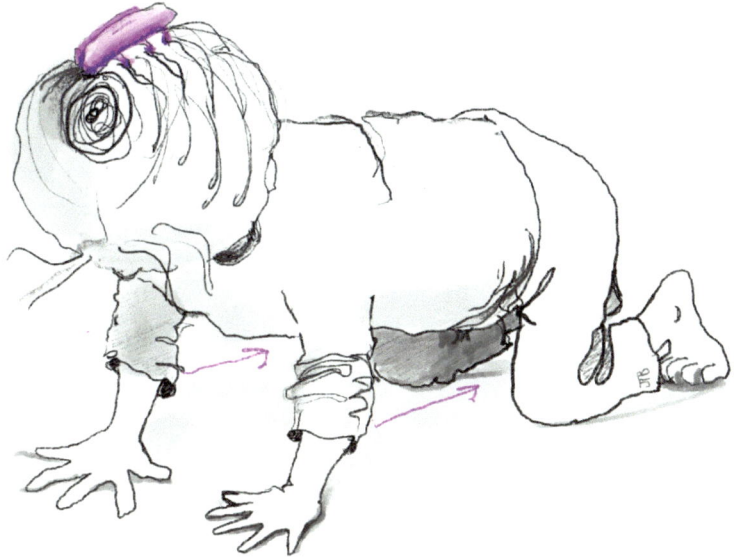

Figure 106 Refine 1.2.

▸ *Practitioner note: If working with a client, ask their permission to place one hand on their sternum, under the collar bones, offering slight upwards support (as subtle resistance) as they bend the elbows and lower towards the ground.*

▶ *Variation 1:* The next time the chest is lowered downward, towards the ground, pause there and once again explore protraction and retraction of the shoulder blades in the lowered position. This added intensity (through the lowered positioning) helps to find further refinement in the movement of the shoulder blades. Push down into the ground, through the handprint, to come up when ready.

▶ *Variation 2:* The next progression is to take the hands further forward, applying pressure to the outside part of the heels of the hands. (This is the base of the little finger, rather than the base of the thumb.) Move from the pelvis towards the hands to shift the weight forwards. Come into a diagonal line from the crown of the head to knees. In this new position, explore retraction and protraction of the shoulder blades. Then add elevation and depression (up and down movements) of the scapulae.

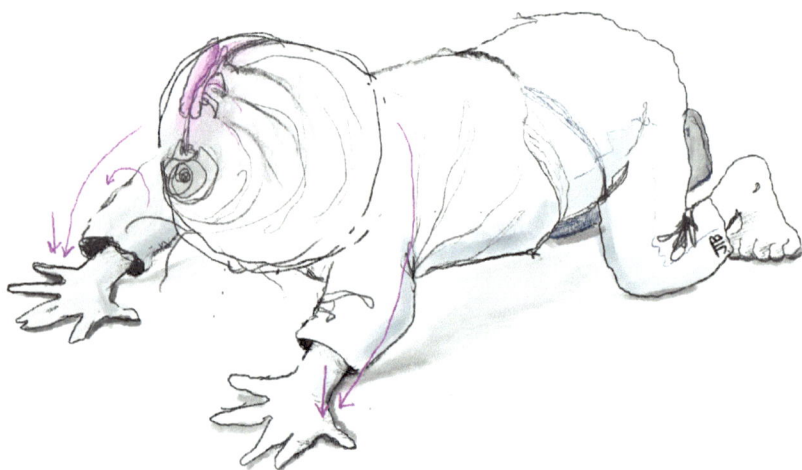

Figure 107 Refine 1.3.

▶ *Variation 3:* Apply a bend to the elbows in this more extended position, being careful not to collapse the spine between the shoulders. The elbows can either point outwards to the sides or backwards towards the tail. The key is to avoid collapsing into the elbows or shoulders. Explore scapula movements of retraction and protraction, elevation, and depression. When ready, gently push through the hands (outside heels of the hands and little fingers) to bring the torso back. Repeat the movement again if there is no feeling of fatigue, before taking a mini break.

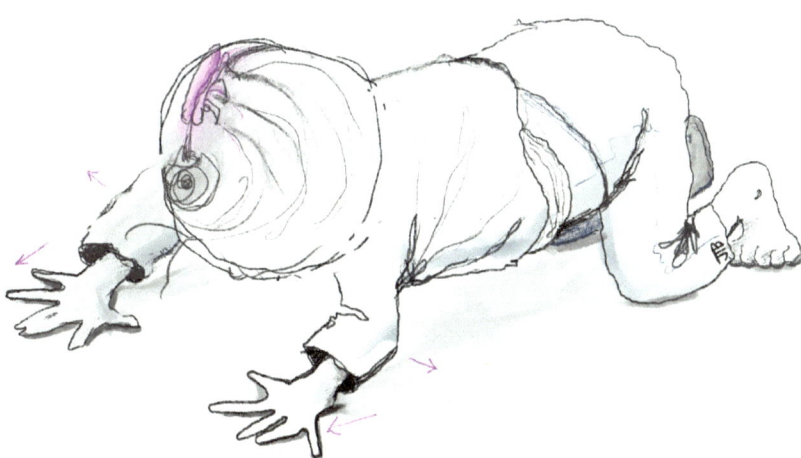

Figure 108 Refine 1.4.

Moderation: If knees are sore, or this is too tricky at first, an excellent moderation is to do exactly this sequence in kneeling, sitting, or standing using the wall, rather than the floor, to press through the arms and shoulders. Ideally, a complete beginner would start at the wall and progress to the floor, unless the floor is not accessible for them.

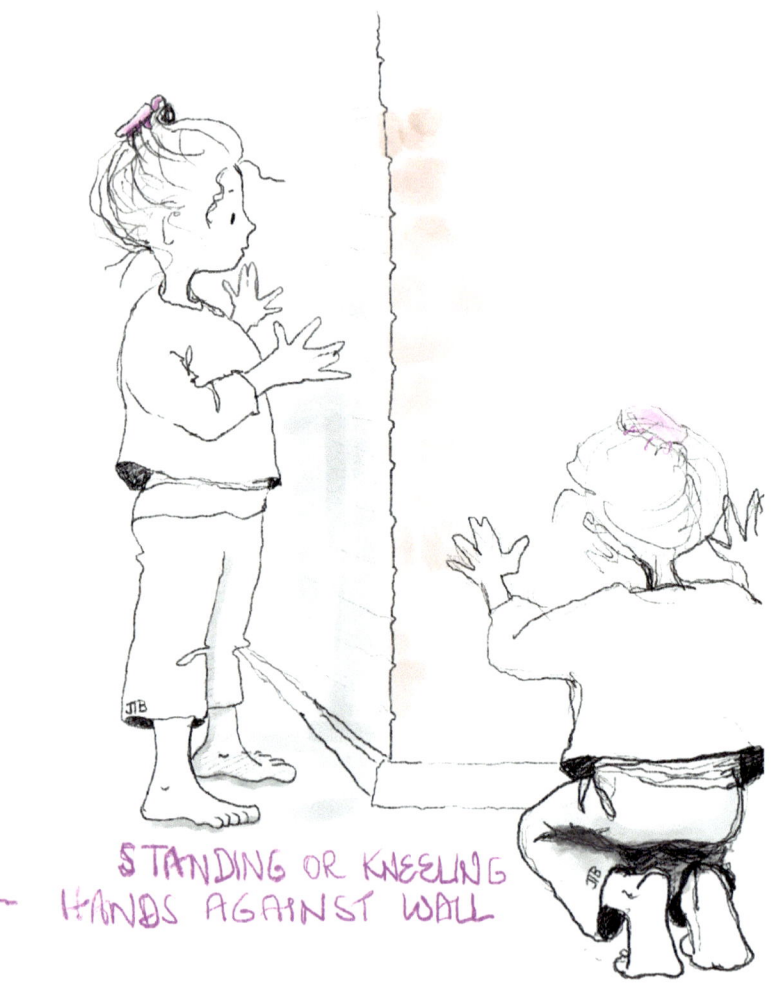

STANDING OR KNEELING
— HANDS AGAINST WALL

Figure 109 Refine 1.5.

Refine 2: semi supine poise

Purpose: Finding poise whilst playing with load, rhythm, direction, and weight distribution.

Support: Stability balls and resistance band.

Timing: As this sequence builds in intensity, take the time to establish refinement at every stage. Play with rhythm and fluidity, moving forwards, backwards, and in rotation.

Sequence:

▸ Come to a seated position with the knees bent and the feet on the ground in front and place the stability ball behind the lower back at the sacrum and the floor. Recline into the ball whilst resting the arms on the front of the thighs, finding a sense of supported balance from the ball pressing back into the lower lumbar spine. Spend a moment finding comfort and stability with the ball.

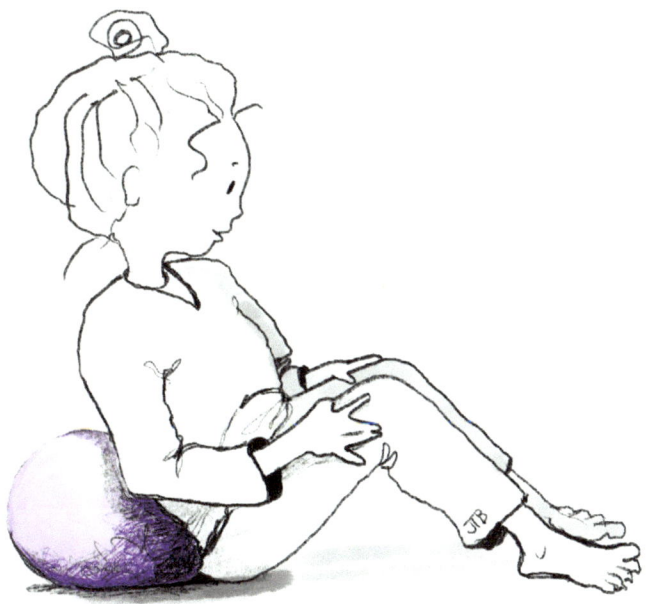

Figure 110 Refine 2.1.

▸ Explore arching the body backwards over the ball, whilst keeping the arms rested and not moving the feet or legs. If this brings on shaking or tremors, stop; this is the neurology letting you know that this particular movement is too demanding at this stage. That is important information. Practise it again another time, or try it earlier in the next practice.

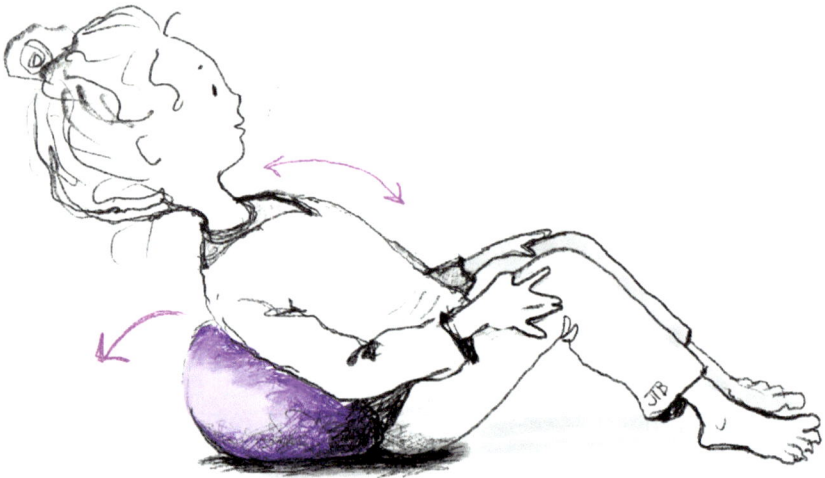

Figure 111 Refine 2.2.

▸ To support the body and help refine the movement, use additional props by taking another stability ball between the knees and holding each end of a resistance band in each hand, wrapping it around the back underneath the armpits. Pulling the band forward with the arms whilst leaning back, helps to find the appropriate tension required to feel supported. This is often enough at the early stage of practice, to help the body feel secure and prevent the tremors that indicate it is too demanding.

▸ Ease the body backwards and forwards, finding a flow and rhythm to the movement. If using the stability band, feel into the oppositional forces of the arms reaching forward while leaning the spine backwards (into the appropriately tensioned band). Then to bring the torso forwards, the shoulder blades draw back and in towards the spine.

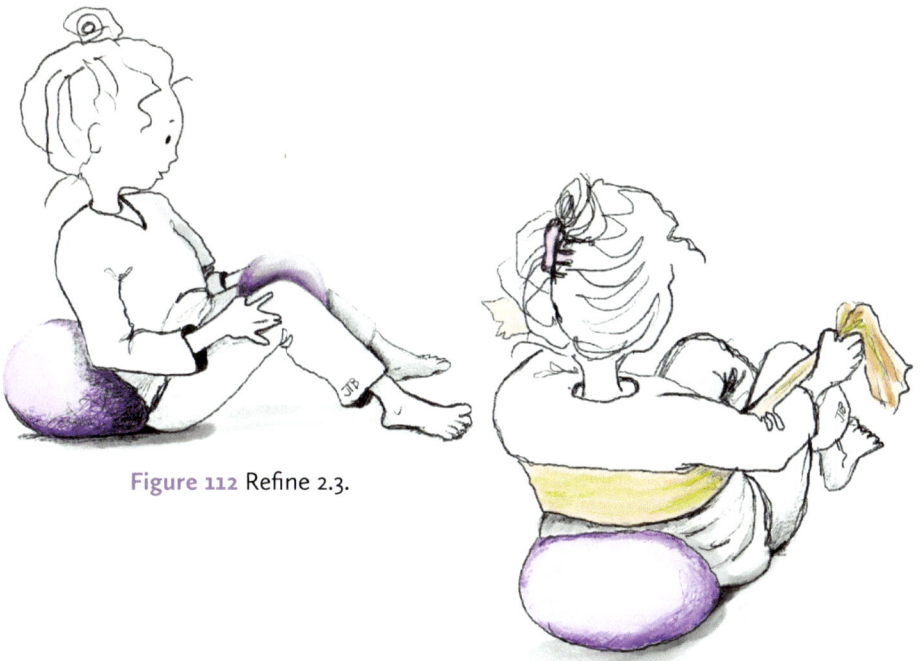

Figure 112 Refine 2.3.

Figure 113 Refine 2.4.

▸ *Variation 1:* The next progression of intensity, once this becomes fluid and relatively easy (which can take several practices, it is worth being very patient), is to remove the supporting ball at the lumbar spine. Repeat the same sequence of moving backwards and forwards without collapsing into the lumbar spine. Once this level is established, it is possible to progress to the next.

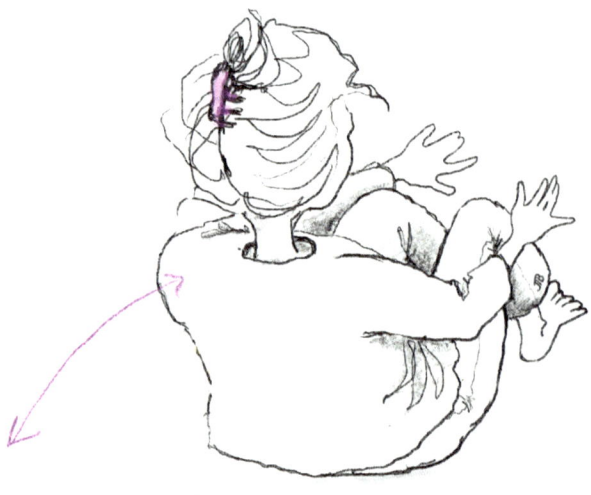

Figure 114 Refine 2.5.

▸ If using the additional resistance band, see if it becomes possible to practise the movement without the band (or the ball behind the sacrum). Once any tremors and vibrations start, go back one stage and add support. If they become less, the body is ready to add intensity and work without the ball or band for support. This is practising refinement, not agility. It is deep, internal balance and poise that becomes progressively easier quite quickly if the body is not over challenged at each stage. Be kind and tune in to the somasense, knowing that there is no need to be in competition with the body's own system. It is a deeply honest practice and responds in small stages and incremental accumulation of poise.

▸ *Variation 2:* This time the theme is to add some load to the movement. Bring one hand to the forehead and one hand to the chest while moving forward. Then reach both arms out in front, to assist when moving back. Then reverse the hand position by swapping the hand on the forehead, with the hand on the chest and reach both hands forward to lean back. Have fun with finding rhythm to these playful sequences, while maintaining integrity at the base. If the legs tremble or the feet come off the floor, restore the ball at the sacrum/lumbar spine and increase the support (i.e., with the resistance band). It gradually becomes easier over time as the somasense gets used to the poise.

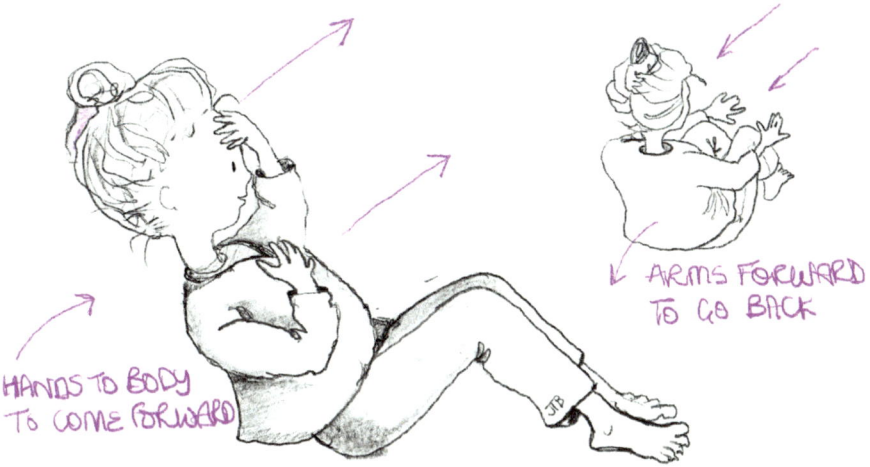

ARMS FORWARD
TO GO BACK

HANDS TO BODY
TO COME FORWARD

Figure 115 Refine 2.6.

▶   *Variation 3:* The final progression is to bring rotation into the movement. While leaning back, offer one hand out to the side, bringing it back the way it came when moving forward, and do the same on the other side, continuing to loop the movement, rotating as the torso comes forward and back, without losing the angle at the hip. Practise this with the ball at the sacrum, then without, to find the rhythmical movements and balance with the changes and variations, as the intensity increases.

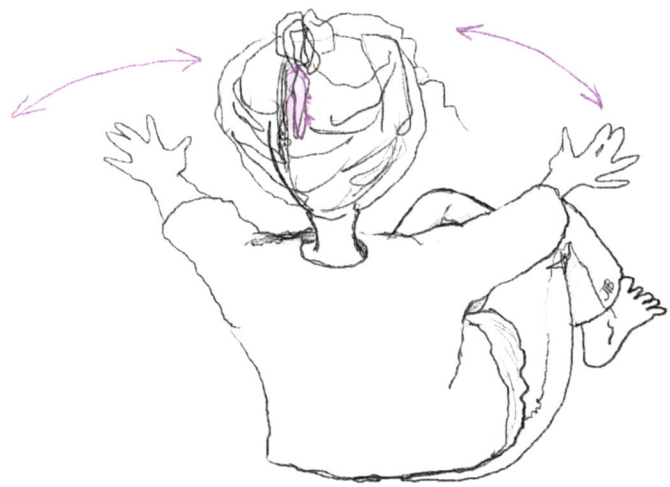

Figure 116 Refine 2.7.

▶ *Variation 4:* To play with additional intensity, take the opposite foot (to the direction of rotation) off the ground, then return it to the ground moving back. Then repeat on the other side. Go slowly to stay attentive to the refinement of the movement. It is helpful to synchronize the breath with the movement, inhaling forward and exhaling back when this more advanced stage is reached.

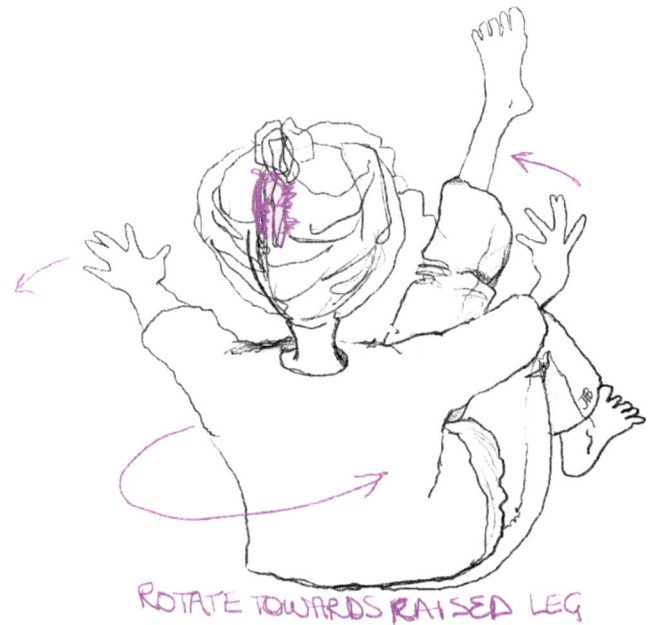

ROTATE TOWARDS RAISED LEG

Figure 117 Refine 2.8.

Refine 3: from supine to side-lying

Purpose: Exploring tensional and oppositional forces to move from supine to side-lying.

Support: The ground, and a stability ball.

Timing: Move slowly to reinforce a sense of resistance and tensional forces through the body to move throughout the sequence with control and grace. Let the quality of the breath and tone of the myofascial matrix guide the repetitions. When the breath and body start to feel fatigued, it's time to stop.

Sequence:

▸ Lie fully supine on a comfortable surface. Float the head slightly off the ground. Gently rock the head from side to side, then rotate left to right. Rest the head back on the floor. Practising this regularly helps develop an active head and cervical spine position so it's dynamically related to the rest of the torso and spine. If head on the ground causes the neck to be arched back, prop with a small towel or another semi-inflated small stability ball.

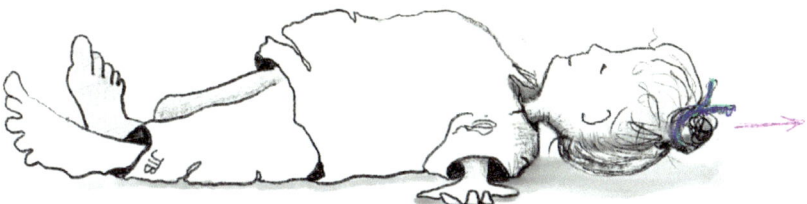

Figure 118 Refine 3.1.

▸ Take the stability ball with both hands, raise the arms up above the body, taking the hands holding the ball back over the head and then forward towards the pelvis. Find a rhythm to the movement, feeling the compliance of the ribs as they respond to where the arms are in space. These can be sensed moving and shifting on the mat as the arms arc the ball.

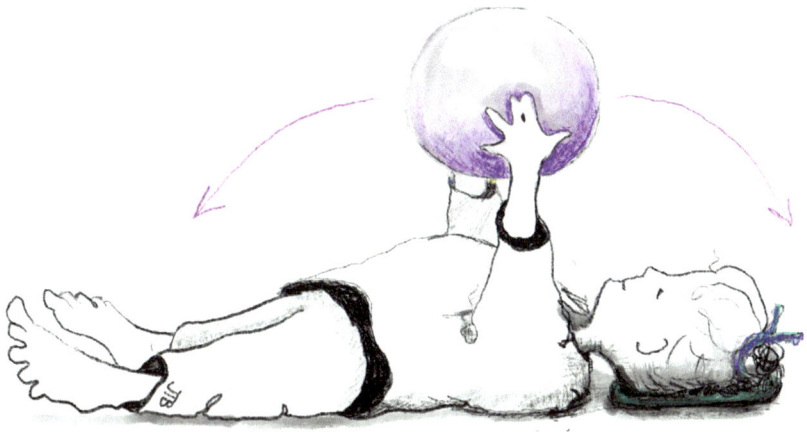

Figure 119 Refine 3.2.

▶ *Variation 1:* Pause the next time the arms are over the head. Hold the position for a few seconds.

▶ *Practitioner note: If working with a client, inform them that gentle pressure will be applied to the ball and invite the client to match the resistance with their entire body. Invite the client to explore movement of their ribs. They can sense gliding the rib cage in an anterior and a posterior tilt, avoiding locking the ribs and 'dropping' the arms to the ground behind them. It is not passive; this slight resistance keeps an active relationship between the arms and the ribs and the pelvis, through the whole body. Whilst the pressure on the ball is maintained, there should still be movement through the whole torso, gently arching and curling.*

▶ If working alone, it is possible to use a slightly heavier prop (e.g., a sandbag), or work with the imagination to evoke a sense of more compression being applied to the ball and see if the tissues respond to the mental suggestion. It requires slightly more poise to find balance and somasense of force distribution through the whole body.

▶ While breathing into this shape and meeting the resistance, seek a sense of the arms, head, cervical, thoracic, and lumbar spine, and legs as one continuity. Feel the continuity and wholeness of the myofascial matrix throughout the 'arc' formation with the ball.

▶ *Variation 2:* The next progression is to continue holding the ball behind the head, imagining that it is very heavy, so that it creates a tensional response through the whole body. On the inhale, lift the right leg slightly off the ground, feeling the left leg press down to support, taking the right leg across the midline, spiralling the body to land gently (and controlled) on the left side, whilst maintaining the contact with (and position of) the ball beyond the crown.

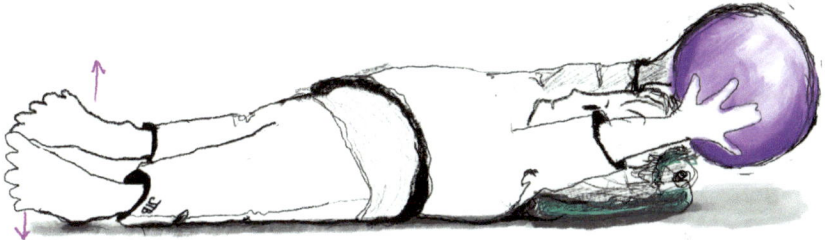

Figure 120 Refine 3.3.

▶ Establish the side-lying position, rolling slightly toward the left side. Exhale with the hands still held beyond the head, reaching away from the navel, and the legs appropriately stiffened, growing out from the lumbar spine. It can be easier to hold both legs slightly off the floor, even if only for a few seconds. Find balance and poise in this side lying position. Avoid dropping the head onto the arm, seeking to hold a long centre through the spine, including the neck and head. Begin with legs on the floor to support the body, gradually progressing to taking the left leg up slightly, to support the right leg from below.

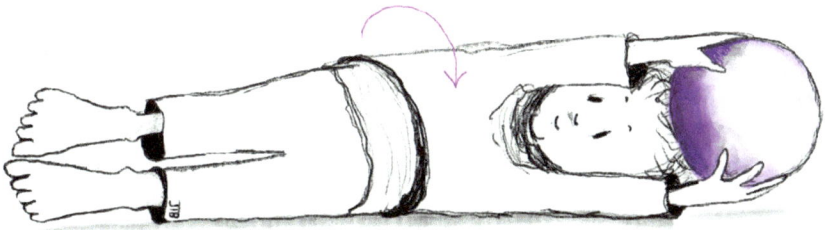

Figure 121 Refine 3.4.

▸ To return to supine position, take the right leg forward (folding at the hip) beyond the left leg in order to stabilize and counterbalance it, while rotating the body slowly back, rolling onto the back again, gradually moving back towards the floor. Avoid collapsing back and dropping into the supine position on the back. This is another example of controlled deceleration. Keep the right leg crossed over the front of the left to counterbalance this movement as the gradual deceleration returns the body to supine. Let the right leg slowly return to the ground once the torso is supine and established on the floor. Rest!

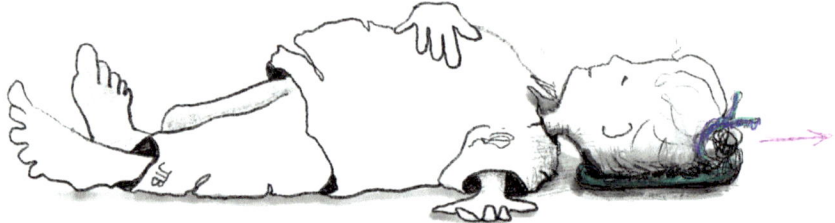

Figure 122 Refine 3.5.

▸ Repeat the entire movement and explore it to the other side, initiating rotation with the left leg, to lie on the right side. Smooth transition and poise through all these changes, using the whole body *experiencing itself as a whole* is the gift of this series. It is myofascial magic in action. Accumulating this ability is like storing treasure. The body can draw on it like a reserve, putting free energy in the myofascial bank! Enjoy.